ASAM PATIENT PLACEMENT CRITERIA:

SUPPLEMENT ON PHARMACOTHERAPIES FOR ALCOHOL USE DISORDERS

ASAM PATIENT PLACEMENT CRITERIA: SUPPLEMENT ON PHARMACOTHERAPIES FOR ALCOHOL USE DISORDERS

EDITOR-IN-CHIEF
Marc J. Fishman, MD

EDITORS
Gerald D. Shulman, MA, FACATA
David Mee-Lee, MD
George Kolodner, MD
Bonnie B. Wilford, MS

Wolters Kluwer Health | Lippincott Williams & Wilkins

Philadelphia • Baltimore • New York • London
Buenos Aires • Hong Kong • Sydney • Tokyo

Acquisitions Editor: Lisa McAllister
Product Manager: Tom Gibbons
Manufacturing Manager: Benjamin Rivera
Vendor Manager: Alicia Jackson
Marketing Manager: Brian Freiland
Cover Designer: Theresa Mallon
Production Service: Maryland Composition Co., Inc/ASI

Wolters Kluwer Health
Two Commerce Square
2001 Market Street
Philadelphia, PA 19103 USA
LWW.com

Printed in China

Library of Congress Cataloging-in-Publication Data

ASAM patient placement criteria : supplement on pharmacotherapies for alcohol use disorders / [edited by] Marc Fishman. — 1st ed.
p. ; cm.
Supplement to the ASAM patient placement criteria, rev. 2nd ed. (ASAM PPC-2R), published by the American Society of Addiction Medicine in 2001.
Includes bibliographical references and index.
ISBN 978-0-7817-9122-9
1. Alcoholism—Chemotherapy—Standards. I. Fishman, Marc (Marc J.) II. American Society of Addiction Medicine. III. ASAM patient placement criteria for the treatment of substance-related disorders. IV. Title: Patient placement criteria. V. Title: Supplement on pharmacotherapies for alcohol use disorders.
[DNLM: 1. Alcohol-Related Disorders—drug therapy. 2. Patient Selection. WM 274 A798 2010]
RC564.7.A83 2010
616.86'1061—dc22

2009033478

To purchase additional copies of this book, call our customer service department at (800) 638-3030 or fax orders to (301) 223-2320. International customers should call (301) 223-2300.

Visit Lippincott Williams & Wilkins on the Internet: at LWW.com. Lippincott Williams & Wilkins customer service representatives are available from 8:30 am to 6 pm, EST.

10 9 8 7 6 5 4 3 2 1

CCS0310

The Editors would like to dedicate this book to our families, who put up with all our time away from them while we worked on it.

ACKNOWLEDGMENTS

The Editors acknowledge with gratitude the contributions of:

- The patients who have taught us so much through their struggles with the terrible illness of addiction, and whose recoveries are testaments to therapeutic optimism;
- The physicians, nurses, counselors, and therapists who work tirelessly in our field to help guide patients toward recovery; and
- Our colleagues, who have provided valuable input and contributed to our thinking on this subject.

CONTENTS

ASAM PATIENT PLACEMENT CRITERIA:

SUPPLEMENT ON PHARMACOTHERAPIES FOR ALCOHOL USE DISORDERS

CHAPTER 1

Introduction

OVERVIEW

The treatment of patients who have alcohol use disorders requires an understanding of many variables, including a complete assessment of the patient's individual medical, psychiatric, environmental, and social issues, as well as knowledge of the uses and limitations of a variety of pharmacologic and nonpharmacologic interventions. All therapies must be individualized to each patient's needs and adjusted to reflect his or her response to treatment. The American Society of Addiction Medicine (ASAM) *Patient Placement Criteria, Second Edition–Revised* (PPC-2R), as well as this Supplement to the Criteria, are designed to assist clinical staff in using the variables to provide timely, appropriate, and effective care.

Alcoholism and Its Treatment

About 3 in 10 U.S. adults drink at a level that increases their risk for medical, psychiatric, and social problems. Of these heavy drinkers, about 1 in 4 meet the criteria for alcohol abuse or dependence—medical disorders that are associated with more than 100,000 deaths from alcohol-related diseases and injuries each year (Harwood, 2000).

Until recently, structured treatment programs based on Twelve Step principles have been the mainstays of treatment for alcohol dependence, with pharmacologic treatments playing a largely adjunctive role. Still, even the best behavioral programs have had a high rate of relapse (O'Brien, 2005).

A growing body of evidence that has emerged over the past decade supports a more central role for medications in the treatment of alcohol dependence. American physicians now have a choice of several different medications—disulfiram (Antabuse®), naltrexone (Revia®, formerly called Trexan and Depade®), acamprosate (Campral®), and extended release, injectable naltrexone (Vivitrol®)—for this indication. Taken together, these medications represent a major advance in the choice of treatments available, as well as in our ability to individualize treatment to the needs of individual patients and thus to improve outcomes.

Almost all studies confirm that medications are most effective when they are part of a comprehensive approach that also incorporates psychosocial therapies (Anton et al., 2006; Carroll, Rounsaville, & Gawin, 1991; Crits-Christoph et al., 1999; Project MATCH Research Group, 1997; Volpicelli, Pettinati, McLellan, & O'Brien, 2001). Such a comprehensive approach is more likely than single-modality approaches to effectively address the multifaceted aspects of alcohol use disorders. Moreover, none of the accepted psychosocial or self-help approaches conflicts in any way with the use of medication to reduce the risk of relapse (O'Brien, 2005).

The course of addiction can be so devastating that the clinician should consider all appropriate therapies to improve the likelihood of a successful outcome for the patient (O'Brien, 2005).

Treatment Planning Using the ASAM Criteria

The *ASAM PPC-2R*, published by the American Society of Addiction Medicine in 2001 (Mee-Lee, Shulman, Fishman, Gastfriend, & Griffith, 2001), are the criteria in widest use today, having been adopted by public and private treatment programs, many State Alcohol and Drug Authorities, managed care organizations, third-party payers, and the U.S. Department of Defense. The ASAM Criteria represent an organized method for integrating the array of services required to meet the needs identified in a multidimensional assessment. They are characterized by six features: (1) clinical assessment with particular attention to risk, (2) individualized treatment planning, (3) facilitation of ready access to services, (4) attention to multiple treatment needs, (5) ongoing reassessment, and (6) modification of the treatment plan in response to reassessment.

Functionally, the criteria are used to match interventions, services, and treatment settings to each patient's particular problems and evolving treatment needs. The ASAM Criteria advocate for individualized, assessment-driven treatment and the flexible use of services across a broad continuum of care.

The criteria also advocate for a system in which treatment is readily available, because patients are lost when the treatment they need is not immediately available and readily accessible. By expanding the criteria to incorporate various levels of outpatient care, especially for those in early stages of readiness to change, the ASAM Criteria have helped to reduce waiting lists for inpatient treatment and thus have improved access to services for all patients.

The ASAM Criteria also embody a philosophy that effective treatment addresses the multiple needs of each patient, rather than focusing solely on his or her alcohol or other drug use. This is based on evidence that, to be effective, treatment must address any associated medical, psychological, social, vocational, environmental, and legal problems. Through six assessment dimensions, the ASAM Criteria underscore the importance of multidimensional assessment and treatment.

The ASAM Criteria are as objective, measurable, and quantifiable as possible, yet certain aspects of the criteria require subjective interpretation. In this regard, the assessment and treatment of substance-related disorders is no different from other medical disorders in which diagnosis, assessment, and treatment involve a mix of objectively measured criteria and experientially based professional judgment.

THE PURPOSE OF THE SUPPLEMENT

Responding to Developments in the Field

Several recent developments provided the impetus for this Supplement to the ASAM Patient Placement Criteria. The addiction field is the beneficiary of a wealth of recent research findings that are directly applicable to clinical practice in addiction treatment. These include the ongoing development and availability of pharmacologic interventions for substance use disorders, as well as for co-occurring medical and psychiatric disorders that have the potential to complicate addiction treatment and recovery.

As responsible clinicians, it is our task to employ the most current, evidence-based strategies to help our patients with substance use and co-occurring disorders move toward recovery. It is for this reason that ASAM, in exercising its responsibility to keep the Criteria as current as possible, decided to develop this *Supplement on Pharmacotherapies for Alcohol Use Disorders*.

The Supplement moves in the direction of best practices in assessing the nature and severity of patients' problems and engaging the full range of pharmacologic and nonpharmacologic therapies to appropriately address those problems. Wherever possible, the recommendations contained here reflect the latest research findings and the clinical experience of recognized experts in the diagnosis and management of substance use disorders.

Rationale for Pharmacotherapy for Alcohol Use Disorders

Why would ASAM choose pharmacotherapy (or medication assisted treatment [MAT]) for alcohol dependence as the topic for its first PPC supplement? By highlighting the advances in this area as an example, we hope to illustrate the use of the broad and increasingly expanding set of tools available to practitioners. The hope is that by using all of the tools at our disposal, we can assist patients to abstinence and then to recovery. An analogy to unicycles, bicycles, and tricycles might help explain this.

Earlier treatment for alcoholism in the modern era consisted exclusively of psychosocial interventions modeled on the philosophy and methods of the Twelve Steps of Alcoholics Anonymous. Early patients underwent "*re*habilitation," that is, they had already acquired the skills to function effectively, but their drinking interfered with the application of these skills. Later, as the field broadened its scope, patients referred to treatment presented with much greater complexity and pathology, and often these patients required "habilitation," with treatment focused on acquisition of skills to function effectively for the first time. Even as the repertoire of additional evidenced-based practices grew, with the expansion of available psychosocial counseling treatments (e.g., cognitive behavioral therapy [CBT], motivational enhancement therapy [MET], Twelve Step facilitation, etc.), successful treatment outcome has been considerably less than desired by providers, payers, and the patients themselves. The use of counseling treatments alone was like riding a unicycle—very difficult to do, with many falls while learning, and not successful for everyone.

It became clear that without additional supports, even the best counseling treatments would be limited in effectiveness. Over time the field has expanded its set of tools to include a broad array of necessary habilitative interventions, previously outside the scope of traditional treatment. These additional tools are typically additional psychosocial interventions used to improve life skills and functioning broadly, and to overcome barriers to counseling and other more traditional treatments. For large numbers of patients, problems with their living conditions, housing, education, employment, job skills, childcare, and transportation create obstacles to recovery that many of them cannot overcome. Interventions addressing these problems, often encompassed under the term recovery support services (RSS), are coupled with counseling and give even more people a chance at sobriety and success. To use the cycling analogy, the field has added the support of two wheels instead of only one, and many more people can ride a bicycle than can ride a unicycle. But, even so, outcomes for alcoholism treatment fall short of expectations.

Increasingly, our appreciation of addiction as a chronic, relapsing disorder reflects scientific advances in our understanding of the structure and function of the brain, the genetics of addiction, and the pharmacology of motivation and behavior. To the extent that pharmacotherapies impacting on biological mechanisms of addiction can reach a wider number of patients or give additional assistance to those partially responsive to psychosocial treatments, we can add a third stabilizing wheel to the bicycle in our analogy. MAT is designed not to replace but to augment psychosocial treatments, such as counseling and RSS. It is a major contribution to the repertoire of alcohol treatments that medications can reduce the likelihood of drinking (whether by aversive conditioning, by reducing positive reinforcement and craving, or by reducing abstinence-related discomfort). To the extent that medications can assist in reducing or stopping drinking, they may help in the attainment and maintenance of sobriety, and they may also increase the likelihood of success of other interventions and change processes.

The broadening of our repertoire of available treatments gives rise to interesting debates and controversies about outcomes and the measures of success. For example, the increasing incorporation of readiness to change as a staging system for treatment matching, and the adoption of MET as a counseling strategy, leads to thinking about improvement more as a heterogeneous, dimensional process, rather than a uniform categorical condition. Patients in a Preparation stage of change, who are attempting to stop drinking with partial but not complete success, are presumably better off than those in a Precontemplation stage who are making no such attempts. Additionally, while full abstinence remains our gold standard, it helps patients for us to understand that its achievement may be gradual as part of the journey toward recovery. While full abstinence remains the appropriate target for treatment, reductions in use short of full abstinence are associated with improvements in psychosocial function, and these are outcomes that are also partial successes, and well worth achieving.

It is important for clinicians to convey to patients and their families what can and cannot reasonably be expected from pharmacotherapies. Any inclinations to overvalue new medications can lead to disappointment and possibly subsequent underutilization. On the other hand, inclinations to dismiss medications entirely as imperfect can lead to unnecessary barriers to recovery. Neither any medication nor any psychosocial treatment for alcoholism has proven to be a magic bullet. Without definitive or universal treatments, we continue to build on our repertoire of treatments that produce dimensional results and succeed with subgroups of patients. These incremental advances are reasons for optimism. We need to reach out for and incorporate every useful tool, and work to learn more about their differential utility. Presumably a balance between medications and psychosocial interventions will lead to the most effective treatment. The availability of three wheels in our tricycle analogy gives us multiple possible points of stability, hopefully each adding cumulative synergies to the others.

The Process of Creating the Supplement

One of the challenges in creating this Supplement has been to resolve the dissonance between two competing goals: (1) to develop a comprehensive document that reflects the most current evidence and employs input from experts in the field, and (2) to move quickly to help clinicians effectively use the evidence-based interventions now available. ASAM's leadership and the Criteria

Drafting Committee resolved the dilemma by developing a subset of the full ASAM Criteria for use in the Supplement. This subset consists of Dimension 1 (Acute Intoxication and Withdrawal Potential) and Dimension 5 (Relapse, Continued Use, or Continued Problem Potential).

Source of Funding

ASAM received support for publication of the Supplement in the form of an unrestricted educational grant from Forrest Laboratories, Inc., and Cephalon/Alkermes, Inc. Neither Forrest nor Cephalon/Alkermes or any other pharmaceutical manufacturer had a role, direct or indirect, in the development of the Supplement or the nature of its contents.

Avoiding Conflicts of Interest

The Editors of the Supplement were sensitive to the need to manage any potential conflicts of interest, which always must be considered in documents of this type.

In accordance with policies established by the Accreditation Council for Continuing Medical Education (ACCME), as ratified by the Board of Directors of ASAM, faculty members, course directors, planning committee members, authors and editors, and others in a position to control the content of an educational activity are required to disclose all relevant financial relationships with any commercial interest within the preceding 12 months. If it is determined that a conflict of interest exists as a result of a financial relationship, that conflict must be resolved prior to the individual's participation in the activity.

The Editors of the Supplement have made the following disclosures of any potential conflicts of interest, as well as their sources of income:

- Dr. Fishman discloses salary from and an ownership interest in an addiction/behavioral health treatment program, from federal grants, and from training and consulting in behavioral health. He receives no income from pharmaceutical manufacturers.
- Dr. Kolodner discloses salary from and an ownership interest in an addiction/behavioral health treatment program. He receives no income from pharmaceutical manufacturers.
- Dr. Mee-Lee discloses income from training and consulting in behavioral health. He receives no income from pharmaceutical manufacturers.
- Mr. Shulman discloses income from training and consulting in behavioral health, including a consulting engagement with Alkermes Inc./Cephalon, Inc., which began in April 2008.
- Mrs. Wilford discloses income from consulting with federal agencies and medical organizations. She receives no income from pharmaceutical manufacturers.

Next Steps In Developing the ASAM Criteria

In the decades since ASAM published the first edition of its Patient Placement Criteria, addiction has increasingly come to be recognized as a chronic disorder that involves complex interactions between drug effects and biological (brain mechanisms, genetic vulnerabilities, and developmental maturation) and environmental (substance availability, social, and economic variables) factors. Its treatment thus requires not only long-term intervention, but also a comprehensive approach that addresses psychiatric, medical, legal, and social consequences. Innovations in assessment, treatment, service delivery, policy, and reimbursement all have changed and will continue to change the field. Such changes demand a response from the Criteria.

The Criteria have evolved over time to reflect the current scientific research. For example, since the first edition was published in 1991, the ASAM Criteria have evolved to encourage clinicians and programs to move:

- From unidimensional to more multidimensional assessment;
- From a generalized assessment to a more specific assessment of risk;
- From program-driven to more clinically driven treatment;
- From a fixed length of stay to variable length of service; and
- From a limited number of discrete levels of care to a continuum of care.

The developers expect the ASAM Criteria to continue to evolve as a result of recent research findings and field experience. Therefore it would be a mistake to wait for a "final" set of criteria before adopting and using the *ASAM PPC-2R* or the *Supplement on Pharmacotherapies for Alcohol Use Disorders*. The development of future editions of the criteria should be approached as a work in progress.

REFERENCES

Anton, R. F., O'Malley, S. S., Ciraulo, D. A., Cisler, R. A., Couper, D., Donovan, D. M., et al., for the COMBINE Study Research Group. (2006). Combined pharmacotherapies and behavioral interventions for alcohol dependence: The COMBINE Study: A randomized controlled trial. *Journal of the American Medical Association, 295*, 17, 2003–2017.

Carroll, K. M., Rounsaville, B. J., & Gawin, F. H. (1991). A comparative trial of psychotherapies for ambulatory cocaine abusers: Relapse prevention and interpersonal psychotherapy. *American Journal of Drug and Alcohol Abuse, 17*, 229–247.

Crits-Christoph, P. L., Siqueland, L., Blaine, J., Frank, A., Luborsky, L., Onken, L. S., et al. (1999). Psychosocial treatments for cocaine dependence: National Institute on Drug Abuse Collaborative Cocaine Treatment Study. *Archives of General Psychiatry, 56*, 493–502.

Harwood, H. J. (2000). *Updating estimates of the economic costs of alcohol abuse in the United States: Estimates, update methods, and data.* Bethesda, MD: National Institute on Alcohol Abuse and Alcoholism.

Mee-Lee, D., Shulman, G. D., Fishman, M., Gastfriend, D. R., & Griffith, J. H. (2001). *ASAM patient placement criteria for the treatment of substance related disorders, second edition-revised (ASAM PPC-2R).* Chevy Chase, MD: American Society of Addiction Medicine.

O'Brien, C. P. (2005). Anticraving medications for relapse prevention: A possible new class of psychoactive medications. *American Journal of Psychiatry, 162*, 8, 1423–1431.

Project MATCH Research Group. (1997). Matching alcoholism treatments to client heterogeneity: Project MATCH posttreatment drinking outcomes. *Journal of Studies on Alcohol, 58*, 7–29.

Volpicelli, J. R., Pettinati, H. M., McLellan, A. T., & O'Brien, C. P. (2001). *Combining medication and psychosocial treatments for addiction—The BRENDA approach.* New York: The Guilford Press.

SUGGESTED READINGS

American Psychiatric Association. (2001). *Diagnostic and statistical manual of mental disorders, fourth edition, text revision* (*DSM-IV-TR*). Washington, DC: American Psychiatric Press.

Bodenheimer, T., Lorig, K., Holman, H., & Grumbach, K. (2002). Patient self-management of chronic disease in primary care. *Journal of the American Medical Association, 288*, 2469–2475.

Carey, K. B., Carey, M. P., Maisto, S. A., & Purnine, D. M. (2002). The feasibility of enhancing psychiatric outpatients' readiness to change their substance use. *Psychiatric Services, 53*, 602–608.

Center for Substance Abuse Treatment, (2005). *Substance abuse treatment for persons with co-occurring disorders. Treatment improvement protocol (TIP) series 42.* DHHS Publication No. (SMA) 05-3992. Rockville, MD: Substance Abuse and Mental Health Services Administration.

DiClemente, C. C. (2003). *Addiction and change – How addictions develop and addicted people recover.* New York: The Guilford Press.

Drake, R. E., Essock, S. M., Shaner, A., Carey, K. B., Minkoff, K., Kola, L., et al. (2001). Implementing dual diagnosis services for clients with severe mental illness. *Psychiatric Services, 52*, 469–476.

Horvath, A. O., & Bedi, R. P. (2002). The alliance. In J. C. Norcross (Ed.), *Psychotherapy relationships that work – Therapist contributions and responsiveness to patients* (pp. 37–69). New York: Oxford University Press.

Institute of Medicine. (2001). *Crossing the quality chasm: A new health system for the 21st century.* Washington, DC: National Academy of Sciences.

Institute of Medicine. (2005). *Improving the quality of health care for mental and substance-use conditions: Quality chasm series.* Washington, DC: Institute of Medicine, National Academy of Sciences.

Jacobson, N., & Greenley, D. (2001). What is recovery? A conceptual model and explication. *Psychiatric Services, 52*, 4, 482–485.

Kizer, K. W. (2001). Establishing health care performance standards in an era of consumerism. *Journal of the American Medical Association, 286*, 1213–1217.

Miller, S. D., Duncan, B. L., & Hubble, M. A. (1997). *Escape from Babel – Toward unifying language for psychotherapy practice.* New York: WW Norton & Company.

Miller, W. R., & Rollnick, S. (2002). *Motivational interviewing: Preparing people for change, second edition.* New York: The Guilford Press.

Mueser, K. T., Corrigan, P. W., Hilton, D. W., Tanzman, B., Schaub, A., Gingerich, S., et al. (2002). Illness management and recovery: A review of the research. *Psychiatric Services, 53*, 1272–1284.

National Institute on Alcohol Abuse and Alcoholism. (2007). *Clinician's guide to the treatment of alcohol problems.* Bethesda, MD: National Institutes of Health.

National Institute on Drug Abuse. (2005). *Principles of drug addiction treatment: A research-based guide.* NIH Publication 05-4180. Rockville, MD: NIDA, National Institutes of Health.

Norcross J.C. (2002). *Psychotherapy relationships that work – Therapist contributions and responsiveness to patients* (pp. 11–14). New York: Oxford University Press.

O'Brien, C. P. (2006, May). *Pharmacotherapies in the treatment of alcohol dependence (CME program).* Paper presented at the Annual Medical-Scientific Conference of the American Society of Addiction Medicine, San Diego, CA.

CHAPTER 2

Role of the ASAM Criteria in the Treatment of Alcohol Use Disorders

OVERVIEW

The goals of the ASAM Patient Placement Criteria include helping patients access the most appropriate and highest quality treatment services; encouraging the development of a broad continuum of care; promoting the effective, efficient use of care resources; and helping protect access to and funding for care. The use of placement criteria in treatment planning thus represents far more than a narrow utilization review or case management process.

Effective implementation of the ASAM Criteria requires a shift in thinking toward outcomes-driven case management. Many organizations concerned with addiction treatment need to make this shift, including regulatory agencies, treatment program administrators and staff, and referral agencies (such as courts, probation officers, child protective services, employers, and employee assistance programs) (Heatherton, 2000).

As outcome analysis increasingly drives treatment decisions, the problems of inadequate access to care and treatment funding are more likely to be resolved.

PRINCIPLES EMBODIED IN THE ASAM CRITERIA

The goals of intervention and treatment (including safe and comfortable detoxification, motivational enhancement to accept the need for recovery, the attainment of skills to maintain abstinence, placement in the least intensive but safe level of care, etc.) determine the methods, intensity, frequency, and types of services to be provided. The clinician's decision to prescribe a type and intensity of service, and subsequently to discharge or transfer a patient from a level of care, are based on how that treatment and its duration will influence the resolution of the dysfunction and positively alter the prognosis for the patient's long-term outcome. Thus, in addiction treatment, the treatment regimen frequently extends beyond simple resolution of observable biomedical distress.

Patients demonstrate a response to treatment by evidencing new insights, attitudes, and behaviors. Addiction treatment programs have as their goal not simply stabilizing the patient's condition, but altering the long-term course of the patient's substance use disorder. That course is often composed of many steps, sometimes in a circuitous path. The steps may involve reductions in use, with partial but incomplete functional improvement; relapse and remission; eventually persistent abstinence; and ultimately the internal changes and personal transformations that accompany a more secure recovery.

As noted in Chapter 1, four principles guide the ASAM Criteria: (1) individualized treatment planning; (2) ready access to needed services; (3) attention to multiple treatment needs; and (4) ongoing reassessment and modification of the treatment plan (Mee-Lee, Shulman, Fishman, Gastfriend, & Griffith, 2001).

Individualized Treatment Planning

The ASAM Criteria reflect a commitment to individualized, assessment-driven treatment and the flexible use of a broad continuum of care. Treatment should be driven not only by ongoing assessment but, more importantly, by evidence of progress, with frequent periodic outcomes measurements. Such evidence might include tracking the treatment alliance, tracking progress toward accomplishment of goals, tracking the patient's continuing substance use (if any), tracking mental health symptoms, etc. The tracking and measurement should be conducted in as close to "real time" as practical—in some cases, at every treatment session. Measurement during treatment that assesses the quality of the patient's engagement and the strength of the therapeutic alliance allows for modification of the treatment plan and level of care in response to the patient's progress or lack thereof.

No single treatment is appropriate for all individuals at all times. Therefore, matching treatment settings, interventions, and services to each individual's particular problems and needs is critical to the patient's ultimate success in returning to productive functioning in the family, workplace, and society.

Therefore, treatment should be guided by an individualized treatment plan that is developed in consultation with the patient. Such a plan should be based on a comprehensive biopsychosocial assessment of the patient and, when possible, a comprehensive evaluation of the family and other collaterals. The plan should list problems (such as obstacles to recovery, knowledge or skill deficits, dysfunction or loss), strengths (such as readiness to change, a positive social support system, and a strong connection to a source of spiritual support), priorities (such as obstacles to treatment and risks, identified within the list of problems and arranged according to severity), goals (a statement to guide realistic, achievable, short-term resolution or reduction of the problems), methods or strategies (the treatment services to be provided, the site of those services, the staff responsible for delivering treatment), and a timetable for follow-through with the treatment plan that promotes accountability.

The plan should be written so as to facilitate measurement of progress. As with other disease processes, length of service should be linked directly to the patient's response to treatment (e.g., his or her attainment of treatment goals and degree of resolution of the identified clinical problems).

Ready Access to Needed Services

To be effective, treatment must be readily available and accessible—otherwise, patients can be lost to the system. By expanding the criteria to incorporate more outpatient levels of care (particularly for patients in the early stages of readiness to change), the ASAM Criteria facilitate the use of outpatient motivational enhancement therapies, thereby increasing access to care by reducing waiting lists for more intensive levels of treatment.

Attention to Multiple Treatment Needs

It is important to recognize that an individual who presents for treatment likely has had a problem with substance use for some time, leading to the development or exacerbation of other problems and disorders. Effective treatment attends to all of a patient's service needs, not just to his or her substance use disorder. Thus, treatment must address any associated medical, psychological, social, vocational, or legal problems. Through the six assessment dimensions, the ASAM Criteria address the importance of multidimensional assessment and treatment. This is congruent with *Principles of Drug Addiction Treatment, Second Edition*, published by the National Institute on Drug Abuse (NIDA), which states that "effective treatment attends to multiple needs of the individual, not just his or her drug use" (NIDA, 2009). Nevertheless, it often is necessary to prioritize the response. From a practical standpoint, it is useful to limit the treatment plan to no more than four or five high priority problems at any point in time, because addressing more than this number can be difficult for the patient. Once a problem has been addressed or resolved, it can be removed from the active treatment problem list and the next highest priority problem added to the list.

Ongoing Reassessment and Modification of the Treatment Plan

Each patient's individual treatment needs and service plan must be continually reassessed and modified to address the patient's changing needs. The ASAM Criteria emphasize ongoing reassessment of the problems that prompted the initial treatment plan and placement, with continuing adjustment of the treatment plan as required.

The process of developing individualized treatment is based on a model of continuous assessment leading to placement and continual reassessment to determine whether continued service or transfer/discharge is most appropriate. Figure 2-1 depicts the process.

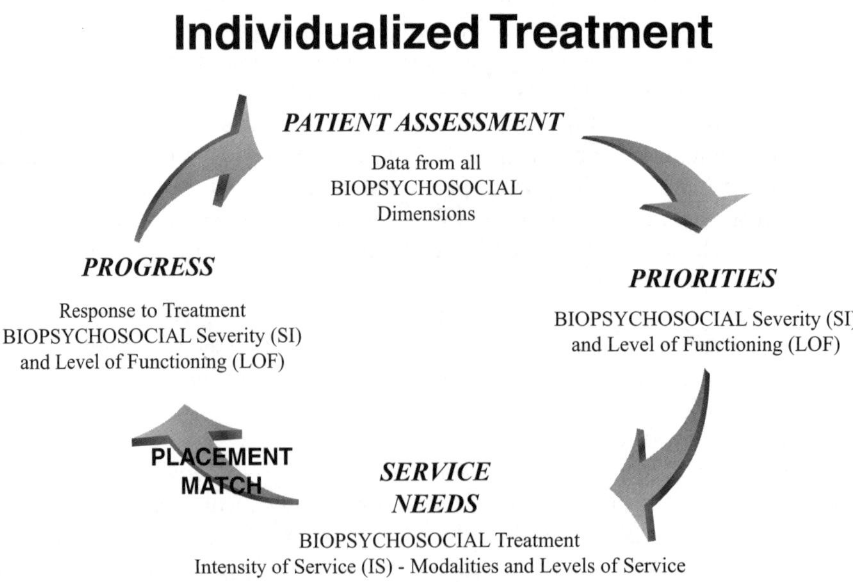

FIGURE 2-1 Developing an individualized treatment plan is a continuous process.

A significant advantage of this approach is its flexibility. For example, consider a case in which a patient in treatment is informed by the state's child protective agency that consideration is being given to removing the patient's children from the home. At this point, the potential loss of custody must be made a very high priority, because the problem threatens to distract the patient from treatment, at the very least.

USING THE ASAM CRITERIA TO MATCH PATIENTS TO TREATMENT

Within the addiction treatment community, at least four models of care have evolved over recent decades, each with a fundamentally different purpose. Although developed at different times, all four models are present today (Mee-Lee, 2001).

1. *Complications-driven treatment* gives only cursory attention to the diagnosis of substance use disorder. Instead of active treatment of the primary alcohol or other drug dependence as the underlying cause, only the secondary complications or sequelae (gastrointestinal, psychiatric, orthopedic, or trauma-related) are addressed. The gastritis or bleeding esophageal varices are controlled, the depression is medicated, fractures are splinted or pinned, but attention to the substance use disorder is superficial or nonexistent. In complications-driven treatment, placement decisions are based on the treatment and outcome of only one aspect of the patient's problem, and progress is measured only in terms of the subspecialty involved. This negatively affects outcome.
2. *Diagnosis, program-driven treatment* recognizes substance use disorder as a primary diagnosis. However, it is the categorical diagnosis that drives the treatment plan rather than the specific needs of the patient. For example, patients are forced to fit into fixed length-of-stay programs, often influenced by the available funding or benefit structure, rather than being placed into a program that meets the patient's specific individual needs. Another example is one in which an *abuse* diagnosis automatically results in referral to an outpatient level of care, while an individual with a *dependence* diagnosis is automatically referred to a residential or inpatient level of care.
3. *Individualized, assessment-driven treatment* emphasizes multidimensional assessment. Problem identification and prioritization are made within the context of the patient's severity of illness and level of function. Treatment services are matched to patient needs over a continuum of care. Results of the ongoing assessment of progress and treatment response influence future treatment recommendations. This continuous quality improvement cycle of assessment, treatment matching, level of care placement, and progress evaluation (as shown in Fig. 2-1) represents a generation of care the addiction treatment field still struggles to implement.
4. *Outcomes-driven treatment* adds the element of outcomes measurement in real time, so that the relationship between patient progress and treatment response is more explicit and concrete. The focus on contemporaneous feedback on issues such as patient engagement, therapeutic alliance, and outcomes affords a greater opportunity for timely modification of the treatment plan. Here, the prioritization of problems and changes in strategies and level of care are augmented by tracking the most salient outcome measures.

However, with outcomes-driven treatment, the promise of matching patients to treatment has yet to be fully realized. For all the rhetoric about *outcomes*—performance measures, accountability, and evidence-based treatment—this generation of addiction treatment is just beginning to be articulated and actualized.

The ASAM Criteria play an integral role in the latter two approaches by providing a multidimensional assessment structure for treatment planning that meets the patient's assessed needs and improves the prospects for a positive outcome. The ASAM Criteria also provide a nomenclature and guidelines to describe an expanded set of treatment options and to promote the use of a wider continuum of services. The criteria thus are intended to enhance the efficient use of limited resources, as well as to increase patient retention in treatment, improve outcome, and prevent dropout and relapse.

The ASAM Assessment Dimensions

The *assessment dimensions* of the ASAM Criteria help to define the severity and character of a patient's disorder in multidimensional terms. The dimensions are intended to assist with the identification of problems and with setting priorities in the treatment plan. The ASAM Criteria identify the following areas of function (dimensions) as the most important in formulating an individualized treatment plan and in making subsequent patient placement decisions. (Note that the information given here is for the adult criteria only.) The prognosis for resolution of problems in the various dimensions depends in part on the difficulty or complexity of each problem and the accuracy of the clinician's assessment of problem severity. It also depends on the degree to which the patient is invested in working on those issues. This interaction between clinician assessment and patient investment forms the basis for the clinician and patient to establish a mutually acceptable treatment plan.

The goals for each problem may need to be reviewed from the standpoint of resolution of the acute crisis and/or alteration of the course of the chronic illness.

Dimension 1: Acute Intoxication and/or Withdrawal Potential

What risk is associated with the patient's current level of acute intoxication? Is the patient so intoxicated as to be nonresponsive? Are symptoms of acute or persistent subacute intoxication likely to be dangerous (as through suicidality, gross disorganization, or aggressiveness)? Is there significant risk of severe withdrawal symptoms or seizures, based on the patient's previous withdrawal history, amount, frequency, and recency of discontinuation of or significant reduction in alcohol or other drug use? Are there current signs of withdrawal? Does the patient have supports to assist in ambulatory detoxification, if medically safe? Has the patient been using multiple substances in the same drug class? Is a withdrawal scale score available?

In the adult ASAM Criteria, detoxification services can be provided at any one of five levels of care. Specific criteria, organized by drug class (alcohol, sedative-hypnotics, opioids, etc.) guide the decision as to which detoxification level is safe and efficient for a patient in withdrawal.

Dimension 2: Biomedical Conditions and Complications

Does the patient have a physical illness other than withdrawal that needs to be addressed because it is exacerbated by withdrawal or is likely to create risk or to complicate treatment? Does the patient have chronic conditions that affect treatment? Is there a need for medical services that might interfere with treatment?

Dimension 3: Emotional, Behavioral, or Cognitive Conditions and Complications

Are there mental disorders or mental health problems that do not present sufficient signs and symptoms to reach the diagnostic threshold? Does the patient have current psychiatric illnesses or psychological, behavioral, emotional, or cognitive problems that need to be addressed because they complicate treatment or create risk? Are there chronic conditions that affect treatment? Do any emotional, behavioral, or cognitive problems appear to be a manifestation of the substance use disorder, or do they appear to be autonomous? Even if connected to the patient's substance use, are they sufficiently severe to warrant specific mental health treatment? Is the patient suicidal and, if so, what is the likelihood that he or she will act on such impulses? Is the patient able to manage the activities of daily living? Can he or she cope with any emotional, behavioral, or cognitive problems? If the patient has been prescribed psychotropic medications, how well does he or she adhere to the therapeutic regimen?

Dimension 4: Readiness to Change

Is the patient actively resisting treatment? Does the patient feel coerced into treatment? How ready is the patient to change? If he or she is willing to accept treatment, how strongly does the patient disagree with others' perception that he or she has a substance use or mental disorder? Does the patient appear to be compliant only to avoid a negative consequence, or is the patient genuinely motivated to address his or her alcohol or other drug use or mental health problem? Where is the patient in the stages of change? Is leverage for change available?

Dimension 5: Relapse/Continued Use/Continued Problem Potential

Is the patient in immediate danger of continued severe mental health distress and/or alcohol or drug use? Does the patient have any recognition or understanding of, or skills in, coping with his or her addictive or mental disorder in order to prevent relapse, continued use, or continued problems such as suicidal behavior? How severe are the problems and further distress that may continue or reappear if the patient is not successfully engaged in treatment? How aware is the patient of relapse triggers, ways to cope with cravings to use, and skills to control impulses to use or impulses to harm self or others? Is the patient likely to remain abstinent or psychiatrically stable, based on his or her history? What is the patient's current level of craving, and how successfully can he or she resist using? If on psychotropic medications, how well does the patient adhere to the therapeutic regimen? If the patient has another chronic disorder (such as diabetes), how well does he or she adhere to the treatment plan for that disorder?

Dimension 6: Recovery Environment

Do any family members, significant others, living situations, or school or work situations pose a threat to the patient's safety or engagement in treatment? Does the patient have supportive friendships, adequate financial resources, and educational or vocational resources that can increase the likelihood of a successful treatment outcome? Are there legal, vocational, social service agency, or criminal justice mandates in place that may enhance the patient's motivation for or engagement in treatment? Are there transportation, child care, housing, or employment issues that need to be addressed? The goals for each problem may need to be reviewed from the standpoint of resolution of the acute crisis and/or alteration of the course of the chronic illness.

Initiating Patient Assessment

Patient assessment begins with data from all biopsychosocial dimensions, which includes a five-Axis DSM and six-Dimension ASAM assessment, as well as any other information available. A problem list is developed from this information, and the identified problems are prioritized according to risk (e.g., incipient delirium tremens [DTs]) and potential obstacles (e.g., lack of transportation and/or child care). In developing this problem list, issues such as severity of illness (SI) and level of functioning (LOF) also are assessed.

Interactions Across Dimensions

The ASAM Criteria function best when individuals are assessed in each dimension independently and also in terms of the interaction across dimensions. A patient's severity and level of function are not determined solely by his or her problems and strengths within a single ASAM Dimension. Instead, severity may increase or decrease because of interactions across Dimensions. For instance, severity in Dimensions 1 through 4 and 6 has an effect on severity in Dimension 5 (Relapse, Continued Use, and Continued Problem Potential). As an example, untreated withdrawal (Dimension 1), an undiagnosed chronic pain disorder (Dimension 2), an unstable psychiatric disorder (Dimension 3), a lack of readiness to change (Dimension 4), or a nonsupportive recovery environment (Dimension 6) all may increase the potential for continued use or relapse. By the same token, good functioning and strengths may decrease severity: a high degree of readiness to change (Dimension 4) and a supportive recovery environment (Dimension 6) may reduce the potential for continued use or relapse.

Assessment of patient severity thus is characterized by the development of a problem or needs list, which then is prioritized by severity. Severity is determined by the degree of risk the patient represents to self or others, or the degree of interference the severity represents in the process of helping the patient access the desired treatment placement. (For example, the absence of transportation or child care may prevent the patient from accessing outpatient treatment.) In developing a severity profile, the clinician should focus on both the patient's history and current status. The final assessment of severity is an expression of both the problems/needs that exist *within* each Dimension as well as the interactions *between* the Dimensions. Table 2-1 presents examples of interactions across Dimensions that have the potential to increase or decrease severity.

Using the Risk Assessment Matrix

Readers familiar with the current ASAM Criteria may notice that the Matrix in this PPC Supplement looks somewhat different from the version presented in the *ASAM PPC-2R* manual (i.e., the Experimental Matrix for Matching Multidimensional Risk with Type and Intensity of Service Needs in Adults [pages 281–312] and Appendix B, the Experimental Matrix for Matching Multidimensional Risk with Type and Intensity of Service Needs in Adolescent [pages 313–339]), though it follows the same basic structure.

In keeping with that structure, as presented here, the Matrix format takes a somewhat different approach to assessment, treatment planning, and placement of the individual with alcohol use disorders from the main Criteria found in the body of the PPC-2R. The Matrix format uses

TABLE 2-1

Examples of Dimensional Interactions That Can Increase or Reduce Severity and Risk

			Dimensional Interactions	
Dimension	*History*	*Current Status*	*Increases Severity*	*Reduces Severity*
Dimension 1: Acute Intoxication/ Withdrawal Potential	History of significant withdrawal symptoms (such as nausea and vomiting; sweats; tremors; seizures; tactile, auditory, and/or visual hallucinations; deliriumtremens)	Current level of intoxication; current withdrawal signs and symptoms (nausea and vomiting; sweats; tremors; seizures; tactile, auditory, and/or visual hallucinations; delirium tremens, fever, anxiety, agitation, depression); quantity of drug used over a given period of time; frequency of use; time elapsed since last use (hours as well as days for substances with a short half-life); recent quantity used compared to capacity; pulse and blood pressure; CIWA-Ar score (for alcohol withdrawal); half-life of substances used; if multiple substances used, potential for drug interactions; ability to cope with withdrawal symptoms	**Dimension 2:** Withdrawal from sedative-hypnotics (e.g., alcohol, barbiturates, benzodiazepines, other sedative hypnotics) complicated by impaired liver function, comorbid neurologic conditions (e.g., a seizure disorder) that could be exacerbated by autonomic nervous system hyperarousal; use or abuse of medications that potentiate the drug from which the patient is withdrawing; pregnancy **Dimension 3:** Use or abuse of psychiatric medications that are metabolized in the liver; pregnancy; psychiatric disorganization that may affect patient adherence to detoxification regimen **Dimension 4:** Lack of readiness to change affecting adherence to detoxification protocols or causing premature discharge from detoxification; lack of readiness to change affecting effectiveness of ambulatory detoxification (as by use of substances overnight or not returning for services the following day)	**Dimension 2:** Absence of a comorbid medical condition **Dimension 3:** Absence of a comorbid psychiatric condition **Dimension 4:** Readiness to change at a level that facilitates adherence to ambulatory detoxification services

(continues)

TABLE 2-1

Examples of Dimensional Interactions That Can Increase or Reduce Severity and Risk *(continued)*

			Dimensional Interactions	
Dimension	*History*	*Current Status*	*Increases Severity*	*Reduces Severity*
		Patients receiving opioid agonist therapy should be checked for drug interactions and possible dose adjustment	**Dimension 5:** Continued use of alcohol, illicit drugs, or nonmedical use of prescription drugs **Dimension 6:** Lack of a supportive recovery environment or transportation for ambulatory detoxification	**Dimension 5:** No continued use of alcohol,illicit drugs, or nonmedical use of prescription drugs **Dimension 6:** A supportive recovery environment and transportation to ambulatory detoxification
Dimension 2: Biomedical Conditions and Complications	History of hypertension; diabetes; gastrointestinal bleeding; advanced liver disease; esophageal varices, especially with a history of a major bleed; HIV/AIDS; hepatitis B or C; other autoimmune diseases; severe polyneuropathy; coronary artery disease; history of stroke combined with current use	Current hypertension, significantly abnormal blood sugar in a diabetic; gastrointestinal bleeding; severe polyneuropathy; pregnancy, particularly with vaginal bleeding; need for regular medical treatment not provided by the addiction treatment provider (e.g., kidney dialysis,	**Dimension 1:** Presence of comorbid medical conditions that could be exacerbated by withdrawal from sedative-hypnotics (e.g., alcohol, barbiturates, benzodiazepines, other sedative hypnotics) with attendant autonomic nervous system hyperarousal (e.g., hypertension complicated by withdrawal from alcohol; presence of medical conditions that could be exacerbated by withdrawal from stimulants (e.g., cocaine, amphetamines)	**Dimension 1:** No withdrawal-related problems.

	of cocaine; chronic pain disorder; history of use of volatile solvents	chemotherapy, physical therapy); chronic pain disorder. Any current comorbid medical problem that would preclude the ability to participate in treatment	**Dimension 3:** Presence of cognitive impairment sufficient to interfere with self-management of a chronic medical condition	**Dimension 3:** Cognitive impairment, if present, is not sufficient to interfere with self-management of a chronic medical condition
			Dimension 4: Lack of readiness to change interfering with the management of a chronic medical condition	**Dimension 4:** Stage of readiness to change is consistent with the management of a chronic medical condition
			Dimension 5: Continued use of hepatotoxic substances in the presence of liver damage; continued use of alcohol when contraindicated by the use of medications for medical conditions (e.g., antiviral drugs); continued use of substances that interfere with the self-management of a chronic medical condition (e.g., diabetes)	**Dimension 5:** Absence of continued use of substances that would complicate a comorbid medical condition or interfere with it self-management
			Dimension 6: Lack of child care or transportation for medical appointments; insufficient financial resources to purchase needed medications	**Dimension 6:** Availability of child care or transportation for medical appointments; adequate finances or other mechanisms to purchase needed medications

(continues)

TABLE 2-1

Examples of Dimensional Interactions That Can Increase or Reduce Severity and Risk *(continued)*

			Dimensional Interactions	
Dimension	*History*	*Current Status*	*Increases Severity*	*Reduces Severity*
Dimension 3: Emotional/ Behavioral Conditions and Complications	Diagnosed Axis I or II disorder, with a history of psychiatric medication nonadherence or ineffectiveness; suicide attempts; family history of suicide; serious self-mutilation, hostile/aggressive acting out; poor impulse control; distractibility; history of ADHD; victimization history; subthreshold mental health problems (e.g., anger management and impulse control problems but insufficient symptoms to meet diagnostic criteria for antisocial personality disorder)	Significant depression, mania, or anxiety; poor or tenuous reality contact; current suicidal/homicidal ideation with plan; poor coping skills; significantly impaired judgment; a GAF score of 45 or less; presence of ADHD interfering with attempts to effectively use treatment; diagnosed unstable Axis I disorder with current psychiatric medication nonadherence or lack of response; current unstable Axis II disorder; diagnostic subclinical Axis I or II disorders; feelings of guilt significant enough to paralyze recovery efforts	**Dimension 1:** Alcohol withdrawal may destabilize psychiatric symptoms (e.g., schizophrenic who has been drinking to "quiet the voices" or a person with bipolar illness who becomes nonadherent with prescribed mood stabilizer resulting in a return to substance use requiring detoxification)	
			Dimension 2: Pressure on coping skills to deal with medical condition (e.g., anxiety about HIV disease or a comorbid chronic pain disorder)	**Dimension 2:** Absence of co-occurring medical conditions that can create emotional stress
			Dimension 4: Lack of readiness to adhere to psychiatric medication directions	**Dimension 4:** Readiness to adhere to the psychiatric medication regimen
			Dimension 5: Continued use of substances that interfere with the effects of drugs for mental health disorders (such as use of alcohol while taking SSRIs for depression)	**Dimension 5:** No use of any substance that could reduce the effects of drugs for mental disorders (e.g., use of alcohol while taking SSRIs for depression)
			Dimension 6: Stressors (DSM Axis IV) that increase pressure on coping skills; homelessness, lack of education,	**Dimension 6:** A positive recovery environment; positive support

			unemployment, lack of positive support system; recovery environment endemic with pressure to use substances or engage in antisocial/criminal behavior; problems with child care and transportation; lack of child care or transportation in general or for mental health treatment appointments; insufficient finances to purchase needed psychiatric medications	system; absence of major stressors about health
Dimension 4: Readiness to Change	Previous treatment history with positive or negative treatment outcomes; attitudes about treatment and self-help groups based on history; awareness of relationship between substance use and problems; history (positive or negative) with treatment or self-help recovery groups; demonstrated ability to adhere to treatment recommendations for other medical conditions (e.g., hypertension, diabetes)	Level of current awareness of relationship between substance use and problems; stage of change on Prochaska and Di Clemente's model (e.g., precontemplation, contemplation, preparation, action, maintenance, relapse, and recycling, termination); current drug craving; internal vs. external motivation; follow through (or lack of) on referral for assessment or treatment; ability to see value in recovery	**Dimension 2:** Lack of success in managing other chronic illnesses (e.g., hypertension, diet compliance for diabetic) **Dimension 3:** History of or current nonadherence with prescribed psychiatric medications low self-esteem; feelings of hopelessness; external locus of control; thought disorder or significant cognitive deficits that interfere with patient's ability to understand the connections between the substance use and resultant problems **Dimension 5:** Continued use in spite of serious adverse consequences	**Dimension 2:** History of adherence to a prescribed medication regimen or other treatment protocols; success in managing other chronic illnesses (such as hypertension) **Dimension 3:** History of adherence to prescribed psychiatric medication regimen; current psychiatric medication adherence; hopefulness about recovery; at least a reasonable level of self-esteem **Dimension 5:** Cessation of use due to serious adverse consequences

(continues)

TABLE 2-1

Examples of Dimensional Interactions That Can Increase or Reduce Severity and Risk *(continued)*

			Dimensional Interactions	
Dimension	*History*	*Current Status*	*Increases Severity*	*Reduces Severity*
			Dimension 6: Lack of positive reinforcement for recovery in the patient's environment; seeing no value in recovery; resistance to change because of negative environmental experience (e.g., abusive parent who gets sober but continues to abuse); absence of external pressures for recovery (e.g., patient consistently enabled by family)	**Dimension 6:** Positive reinforcement in the recovery environment; patient perceives value in recovery; something of value in the recovery environment at stake with continued use (e.g., employment, marriage, freedom, professional license); presence of external pressures for recovery (e.g., family employing "tough love" with adolescent)
Dimension 5: Relapse/ Continued Use/ Continued Problem Potential	Past history of ability to remain abstinent; past relapse history; history of adherence with addiction medication (anticraving or aversive medication)	Source of motivation (e.g., internal vs. external); stage of readiness to change; current use, craving, and understanding that craving does not inevitably result in use; withdrawal; possession of relapse prevention strategies including	**Dimension 1:** Current use of alcohol or other nonprescribed drugs; incomplete withdrawal from psychoactive substances **Dimension 2:** Presence of an acute medical problem (such as pancreatitis) that produces physical pain; a chronic pain disorder; a medical problem that distracts from recovery efforts	**Dimension 1:** Absence of craving associated with current use or withdrawal **Dimension 2:** Absence of pain associated with a medical disorder; absence of a medical problem creating distraction from recovery efforts

	identification of high risk situations and triggers and a PLAN for responding to them without using; pharmacologic responsivity (e.g., positive reinforcement from use and/or negative withdrawal reinforcement)	**Dimension 3:** Presence of a comorbid, poorly managed Axis I or II disorder or Axis I (e.g., anxiety) or Axis II (e.g., impulsivity or poor anger management skills) traits that do not meet DSM diagnostic thresholds (i.e., subclinical); external locus of control	**Dimension 3:** Absence of psychiatric comorbidity; presence of an internal locus of control
		Dimension 4: Patient is not ready to change, or does not understand the connection between substance use and associated problems	**Dimension 4:** Patient is ready to change and understands the connection between substance use and associated problems
		Dimension 6: Absence of a positive social support system; using/abusing social support system; perceiving no value in recovery; social support system encouraging abusive use; support system oppositional/sabotaging; resistance to change because of negative environmental experience (e.g., abusive parent who gets sober but continues to abuse); absence of external pressures for recovery (e.g., patient consistently enabled by family); lack of high school education or GED; unemployed; lack of employment skills; ex-convict; homeless; unsafe housing (e.g., being physically, emotionally or sexually abused)	**Dimension 6:** Presence of a positive social support system; perceived value in recovery; positive environmental recovery experiences; external pressures for recovery (e.g., patient not enabled by family); high school education or GED; employed or with employment skills; safe place to live

(continues)

TABLE 2-1

Examples of Dimensional Interactions That Can Increase or Reduce Severity and Risk *(continued)*

			Dimensional Interactions	
Dimension	*History*	*Current Status*	*Increases Severity*	*Reduces Severity*
Dimension 6: Recovery Environment	Lack of experience with application skills for education or employment; ex-convict; lack of experience developing a positive social support system	Lack of positive social support system; environment in which there is direct or indirect pressure to use (e.g., all friends are users or dealers); opportunity so limited there is little advantage to recovery; illiteracy; lack of education (no high school diploma or GED); unemployed; lack of job skills, housing problems; child care problems; lack of adequate transportation; single parent status; lack of effective parenting skills	**Dimension 3:** Presence of behaviors associated with a co-occurring mental disorder, which create environmental problems (e.g., loss of housing due to atypical behavioral associated with hallucinations in schizophrenia, loss of employment because of criminal behavior associated with antisocial personality disorder) **Dimension 4:** Lack of readiness to change, resulting in poor decisions regarding the recovery environment (e.g., electing to remain in environment with pressures to use when other options exist) **Dimension 5:** A recovery environment that accepts continued use of relapse	**Dimension 4:** Readiness to change a nonsupportive recovery environment **Dimension 5:** A recovery environment that does not accept continued use of relapse

a more quantitative system for assessing risk, thereby enhancing the user's ability to identify areas of concern and to select appropriate interventions as components of a comprehensive treatment plan. It uses a three-column format to emphasize the need to determine the type and modality of services needed (column 2) and only then to determine the appropriate level of care (column 3). This Supplement and its Matrix format are not intended to replace the PPC-2R, but rather to refine and expand the material presented in the PPC-2R as it relates specifically to the treatment of alcohol dependence.

Goal of the Matrix

The primary goal of the Matrix is to promote improved assessment, treatment planning, and placement of patients with substance use disorders (with or without co-occurring disorders) by adopting a more holistic, multidimensional approach that matches the patient's needs to specific treatment services rather than merely to broad levels of care.

To optimize the use of treatment and financial resources, patient care must be individualized rather than driven only by the patient's diagnosis, the availability of certain levels of care or types of treatment programs, or the availability of treatment services reimbursement or funding.

The patient's diagnosis is a necessary but insufficient determinant of service needs. As is true of patients who are diagnosed with cancer, hypertension, or diabetes, it is the severity of the patient's illness and the degree of the patient's impairment—not merely the diagnosis—that determine the patient's specific treatment needs and thus drive the treatment plan. The Risk Assessment Matrix thus reflects the following concepts:

1. *Risk is multidimensional and biopsychosocial.* Addressing a particular patient's risk may require more than one treatment component (e.g., stabilizing a psychosis or detoxifying a patient while also addressing an unstable or abusive living environment).
2. *Risk relates to the patient's history.* For example, the patient whose withdrawal always results in seizures has treatment needs that differ from the patient whose withdrawal involves only mild symptoms of anxiety. Or the patient who in the past has acted on suicidal impulses by attempting to hang himself has needs different from the patient who acted on suicidal impulses by superficially scratching a wrist.
3. *Risk is expressed in current status.* For example, a patient who develops elevated vital signs in response to discontinuation of alcohol use requires different treatment services from a calm patient who is not currently using alcohol or other drugs. Similarly, an actively psychotic patient who is hallucinating needs more intensive services than a patient who is chronically psychotic but currently stable.
4. *Risk involves a degree of change from baseline or premorbid functioning.* For example, a previously outgoing and fully functioning individual who suddenly withdraws from social contact needs more intensive services than does an individual who is chronically withdrawn and barely able to function outside of a supportive living environment.
5. *Risk assessment must integrate the patient's history, changing situation, and current status* into a comprehensive profile of risk.

Determining Service Needs and Level of Care

Once a Risk Rating has been determined in each domain, the Risk Assessment Matrix can be used to determine the patient's service needs and level of care. To use the Matrix format most effectively, the clinician performs a comprehensive assessment of the patient's strengths and problems in each of six dimensions. Once a problem list is created, it is prioritized by severity (e.g., Dimension 2, advanced liver disease in an alcohol-dependent patient), risk (as in Dimension 3, suicidal thought with high lethality), or interference (reflected in Dimension 6, lack of child care or transportation for a patient who appears to be a likely candidate for an outpatient level of care).

In column 1 of the Matrix, each of the prioritized problems is assigned a Risk Rating, ranging from 0 (no or stable problem), to 1 (minimal risk), 2 (moderate risk), 3 (significant risk), or 4 (severe risk). Based on the Risk Rating assigned in column 1, the appropriate services are selected from column 2, as are the modalities for delivering the services and the dose (column 3). For example, if a patient is assessed as being at severe risk for relapse to alcohol use (Dimension 5, Risk Rating 3) in column 1, the services selected from column 2 might include relapse prevention treatment services such as individual and group counseling, as well as initiation of a medication for alcohol dependence (modalities) given daily (dose). In column 3, placement at a particular level of care is determined. It is not unusual for particular service needs and intensities to be met at more than one level of care. Patients should be placed at the least intensive level at which the patient can safely and effectively receive treatment.

The emphasis of the Matrix format is primarily on services and modalities of care and only secondarily on the site at which care is delivered. This is consistent with a continuing emphasis on "unbundling" of services. Each Dimension is initially considered separately from the other Dimensions to allow for independent assessment of all areas of potential concern. Table 2-2 gives an example of this process in Dimension 5, while Table 2-3 gives an example in Dimension 1.

TABLE 2-2

Sample Assessment of a Patient in Dimension 5

Nature of the Problem	
• Risk of relapse to alcohol use	
Severity of the Problem	
• Significant (Risk Rating of 3)	
Services Required	
• Relapse prevention	
Modalities and Dose	
Modality	***Dose***
• Supportive group counseling	5×/wk
• Cognitive behavioral therapy individual counseling	2×/wk
• Intensive monitoring	5×/wk
• Initial medication assessment	ASAP, 1×
• Ongoing medication management	Weekly, then tapering

Placement Considerations

Level II.5 may be most appropriate for the patient's needs in Dimension 5, possibly in combination with Level I outpatient medical office services. However, the patient's needs in other Dimensions may modify the placement decision.

TABLE 2-3

Sample Assessment of a Patient in Dimension 1

Nature of the Problem • Alcohol withdrawal	
Severity of the Problem • Significant (Risk Rating of 3)	
Services Required • Detoxification	
Modalities and Dose	
Modality	***Dose***
• Medical assessment for management of withdrawal	Immediately
• Supportive group counseling	Daily
• Medical management of withdrawal, including pharmacologic therapies	Daily
• Intensive monitoring of progress	Multiple times a day
Placement Considerations Level III.7-D may be most appropriate for the patient's needs in Dimension 1. Alternatively, the patient may be placed at Level II.5-D, if available as a daily medically monitored service, and if adequate overnight support can be provided by the patient's family. Note that other Dimensional needs may modify the placement.	

The next step is to perform a similar assessment of the patient in each of the other Dimensions, as well as for interdimensional interactions. For example, consider a patient who is at significant risk (Risk Rating of 3) of alcohol withdrawal (Dimension 1) and thus requires detoxification services, assessment, monitoring, medication management, and counseling, at an initial dose of 7 days per week, as shown in Table 2-3.

Compliance Versus Adherence

Treatment or medication *compliance* is a term long used in the health care field in general and in the addiction and mental health sectors in particular. *Webster's Dictionary* defines "to comply" as "to act in accordance with another's wishes, or with rules and regulations." By contrast, it defines "adhere" as "to cling, cleave (to be steadfast, hold fast), to stick fast." The term "compliance" is falling into disuse. Significant parts of the health care field have been using "adherence" for some time, which is contributing to a greater focus on collaborative approaches that engage and empower patients.

It is no longer seen as appropriate for a counselor or other professional to develop a plan with which a patient must only *comply*, nor is it appropriate for a physician to prescribe a medication with which a patient must demonstrate only medication *compliance*. Patient engagement and responsibility to change through utilizing available tools is the goal hoped for beyond passive compliance. This is not at all to minimize the critical expertise that physicians (and other clinicians) bring to the doctor–patient relationship, nor to negate the importance of our standard teaching that addiction patients in particular must learn to look outside themselves for sources of assistance. Rather, it is to emphasize a strategic approach to improving patient utilization of that expertise and assistance through attention to alliance and motivation. Stages of change models and motivational enhancement therapies have been shown to be effective in engaging patients and changing their attitudes and behaviors. Over the past 30 years, more than 2000 research papers have been published on the concept of the therapeutic alliance. These findings emphasize the importance of developing the alliance with patients, especially in the early phases of treatment (Center for Substance Abuse Treatment, 2005; DiClemente, 2003; IOM, 2001, 2005; Miller & Rollnick, 2002).

For all the foregoing reasons, the term "adherence" rather than "compliance" is used in this Supplement when referring to the patient's collaboration and participation in treatment.

CARING FOR PATIENTS WITH CO-OCCURRING DISORDERS

When the first edition of the ASAM Criteria was published in 1991, the criteria were designed for programs that offered only addiction treatment services. However, even that early edition acknowledged that some patients come to treatment with medical (Dimension 2) and psychiatric (Dimension 3) disorders that coexist with their substance-related problems. Clinical reality suggests that programs and practitioners who are committed to meeting the total needs of the patients they serve must be able to meet the needs of these "dual diagnosis" patients, now more frequently referred as patients with "co-occurring or comorbid disorders." This concept is particularly relevant today, as the range of patient needs and clinical variability continues to broaden.

Factors contributing to this clinical reality include the increase in substance use and substance-related disorders in younger populations; greater sensitivity to substance use problems in the mental health, welfare, and criminal justice systems; and increased commitment to early intervention in substance use disorders in preference to fragmented services and incarceration later in the progression of the disorder. Another major factor has been the growing body of scientific evidence pointing to the effectiveness of psychiatric medications in treating patients with co-occurring disorders. Greater understanding of the uses and effects of psychosocial and cognitive-behavioral strategies also has heightened awareness of a broadened range of modalities to meet individual needs.

The ASAM Criteria thus address the large subset of individuals who present for treatment with co-occurring Axis I substance-related disorders and Axis I/Axis II mental disorders. Individuals with such co-occurring disorders can be conceptualized as belonging to one of two general categories:

- *Moderate Severity Disorder:* Such persons present with stable mood or anxiety disorders of moderate severity (including resolving bipolar disorder), or with personality disorders of moderate severity but stable (although some persons with severe levels of antisocial personality disorder may be appropriately placed in this group), or with signs and symptoms of a mental health disorder that are not so severe as to meet the diagnostic threshold.

- *High Severity Disorder:* Such persons present with schizophrenia-spectrum disorders, severe mood disorders with psychotic features, severe anxiety disorders, or severe personality disorders (such as fragile borderline conditions) and are unstable.

Individuals whose co-occurring mental disorders best fit within the category of moderate severity disorders are appropriately treated in programs designed to treat primary substance use disorders. Those with concurrent high severity mental disorders, on the other hand, generally are best managed in dual diagnosis specialty programs that can offer integrated mental health and addiction treatment approaches. Some patients may require immediate stabilization of their psychiatric symptoms before they can be engaged in ongoing addiction treatment and recovery. Depending on the severity of their symptoms, such patients may require referral to medical and/or psychiatric services.

Once stabilization has been achieved, the initial placement for recovery services should reflect an assessment of the patient's status in all six dimensions. The principle here is that the highest severity problem (particularly those in Dimensions 1, 2, or 3) should determine the patient's initial placement. Subsequent resolution of this problem creates an opportunity to transfer the patient to a less intensive level of care. Addressing the individual's recovery needs thus may involve a sequence of services across several levels of care (involving a "step down" or "step up" process). For example, a patient who is assessed in Dimension 2 as uncontrolled hypertensive should be placed in a Level III.7 or Level IV program to stabilize his or her medical condition before being transferred to a Level I program for treatment of the substance use disorder. What should be avoided is the notion of "averaging" severity across dimensions to arrive at a placement determination.

Patients whose biomedical or psychiatric disorders are so severe that stabilizing them is the highest priority are most appropriately treated in a medical or psychiatric facility or unit before addiction treatment is initiated.

ASSESSMENT OF IMMINENT DANGER

Imminent danger is defined as the presence of all three of the following elements: (1) a strong probability that certain behaviors will occur (e.g., continued alcohol or drug use or relapse or nonadherence to the use of psychiatric medications); (2) the likelihood that such behaviors will present a significant risk of serious adverse consequences to the individual and/or others (as in a consistent pattern of driving while intoxicated); and (3) the likelihood that such adverse events will occur in the very near future.

If a patient has problems in Dimensions 4 and 5 (such as boundary setting) that require 24-hour supervision and treatment, and without which treatment services cannot be effectively delivered, and/or the individual is in imminent danger, then the addition of room and board would be insufficient to meet the patient's needs. Instead, such a patient requires placement in a residential program that offers clinical staff and services 24 hours a day, so as to respond to the patient's issues that account for the imminent danger. Assessment of risk should guide the decision.

In the Matrix format, each risk description provides both a numerical Risk Rating (on a scale of 0 to 4, indicating increasing severity) and a narrative description of risk in terms of signs and symptoms that indicate the individual's severity and level of function in a particular Dimension.

The risk descriptions and ratings are designed to help staff determine the immediacy and scope of the service plan by describing the types and modalities of services that may be needed. They also indicate the intensity or level of service at which a given patient can be treated with safety and efficacy.

The risk rating numbers correlate with the severity of the patient's problems in the following manner:

- A Risk Rating of 0 indicates *no* problems in that Dimension.
- A Risk Rating of 1 indicates *minimal* problems in that Dimension.
- A Risk Rating of 2 indicates *moderate* problems in that Dimension.
- A Risk Rating of 3 indicates *significant* problems in that Dimension.
- A Risk Rating of 4 indicates *severe* problems in that Dimension.

Step 1

The patient should be assessed to determine whether he or she has immediate needs related to imminent danger, as indicated by a Risk Rating of 4 in any of the six dimensions.

Step 2

If the patient is not in imminent danger, he or she should be assessed separately for the substance use disorder and any co-occurring medical (Dimension 2) or psychiatric disorders (Dimension 3). This assists in identifying his or her medical, psychiatric, and addiction treatment needs and facilitates identifying the kind of treatment program that is most likely to meet the patient's needs.

Step 3

The types of services and modalities appropriate to the patient's level of risk should be identified.

Step 4

The resulting Risk Profile should be used to develop an initial treatment or service plan. A service plan differs from a traditional treatment plan in that the focus is on the assessment of problem severities, types of services and modalities needed, and the least intensive level of care in which the patient's needs can be safely met. The service plan does not address details such as the responsible staff member, the time frame for completion of treatment, or the methods to be used, except as they might relate to placement decisions.

The most appropriate placement is achieved by identifying the level of care at which the various service needs in all relevant dimensions can be provided effectively and efficiently. The appropriate intensity of service, level of care, and setting may be the highest Risk Rating across all the dimensions. Consider, however, that the interaction of needs across all dimensions may require more intensive services than the highest Risk Rating alone.

Step 5

Ongoing decisions about the patient's continued service needs and placement should be made by repeating Steps 1 through 4. Movement into and through the continuum of care should be a fluid and flexible process that is driven by continuous monitoring of the patient's changing Multidimensional Risk Profile.

INABILITY TO ACCESS SERVICES AND OTHER PLACEMENT DILEMMAS

In some situations, services a patient needs may be unavailable. For example, there may be geographic barriers, if services are not available in the patient's geographic area. This might be remedied by concurrent treatment by two service providers, or referral for the less urgently needed service after the primary service have been delivered. In other situations, the service may be available, but not at the indicated level of care.

In some geographic areas, multiple services are available, but they do not represent a true continuum of care, which is characterized by three characteristics: (1) seamless transfer between providers; (2) philosophical congruence among provider belief systems; and (3) the patient never arrives at the next provider before the clinical record. (This is a systems problem, beyond the ability of individuals to repair, but is raised here to alert clinicians to the potential obstacles to patients receiving the care they need in a timely manner.)

There also are financial barriers, as when insurers and benefit managers limit access to care or the duration of that care. In such situations, appropriate care should be sought in the publicly funded treatment system.

Another financial barrier arises when a patient cannot afford to purchase a prescribed psychiatric or antiaddiction medication. A possible resource in such a situation is found in some pharmaceutical manufacturers' patient assistance programs.

REFERENCES

Al-Otaiba, Z., Worden, B. L., McCrady, B. S., & Epstein, E. E. (2008). Accounting for self-selected drinking goals in the assessment of treatment outcome. *Psychology of Addictive Behaviors, 22*, 3, 439–443.

American Psychiatric Association. (2000). *Diagnostic and statistical manual of mental disorders, fourth edition, text revision*. Washington, DC: American Psychiatric Press.

Anton, R. F., O'Malley, S. S., Ciraulo, D. A., Cisler, R. A., Couper, D., Donovan, D. M, et al. (2006). Combined pharmacotherapies and behavioral interventions for alcohol dependence – The COMBINE Study: A randomized controlled trial. *Journal of the American Medical Association, 295*, 17, 2003–2017.

Center for Substance Abuse Treatment. (2005). *Substance abuse treatment for persons with co-occurring disorders. Treatment improvement protocol (TIP) series 42*. (DHHS Publication No. 05-3992). Rockville, MD: Substance Abuse and Mental Health Services Administration.

DiClemente, C. C., Haug, N., Bellino, L., & Whyte, S. (2003). *Psychotherapy and motivational enhancement. Recent Developments in Alcoholism, 16*, 115–132.

Diehl, A., & Mann, K. (2007). Pharmacological relapse prevention in alcohol and tobacco dependence. *Internist (Berl), 48*, 1, 79–84, 86–88.

Donovan, D. M., Anton, R. F., Miller, W. R., Longabaugh, R., Hosking, J. D., Youngblood, M., COMBINE Study Research Group. (2008). Combined pharmacotherapies and behavioral interventions for alcohol dependence (The COMBINE Study): Examination of posttreatment drinking outcomes. *Journal of Studies on Alcohol and Drugs, 69*, 1, 5–13.

Dundon, W. D., Pettinati, H. M., Lynch, K. G., Xie, H., Varillo, K. M., Makadon, C., et al. (2008). The therapeutic alliance in medical-based interventions impacts outcome in treating alcohol dependence. *Drug and Alcohol Dependence, 95*, 3, 230–236.

Garbutt, J. C. (2009). The state of pharmacotherapy for the treatment of alcohol dependence. *Journal of Substance Abuse Treatment, 36*, 1, S15–23.

Gartner, L., & Mee-Lee, D. (1995). *The role and current status of patient placement criteria in the treatment of substance use disorders.* (Treatment Improvement Protocol No. 13). Rockville, MD: Center for Substance Abuse Treatment.

Gastfriend, D., Rubin, A., Sharon, E., Turner, W. M., Anton, R. F., Donovan, D. M., et al. (2003). New constructs and assessments for relapse and continued use potential in the ASAM Patient Placement Criteria. *Journal of Addictive Diseases, 22*(Suppl.1), 95–111.

Godley, M. D., Godley, S. H., Dennis, M. L., Funk, R. R., & Passetti, L. L. (2007). The effect of assertive continuing care on continuing care linkage, adherence and abstinence following residential treatment for adolescents with substance use disorders. *Addiction, 102*, 1, 81–93.

Heatherton, B. (2000). Implementing the ASAM Criteria in community treatment centers in Illinois: opportunities and challenges. *Journal of Addictive Diseases*, 19, 2, 109–116.

Hilton, T. (2007). Pharmacological issues in the management of people with mental illness and problems with alcohol and illicit drug misuse. *Criminal Behaviour and Mental Health, 17*, 4, 215–224.

Institute of Medicine. (2001). *Crossing the quality chasm: a new health system for the 21st century.* Washington, DC: National Academies Press.

Institute of Medicine. (2005). *Improving the quality of health care for mental and substance-use conditions: quality chasm series.* Washington, DC: National Academies Press.

Johnson, B. A. (2008). Update on neuropharmacological treatments for alcoholism: Scientific basis and clinical findings. *Biochemistry Pharmacology, 75*, 1, 34–56.

Johnston, M. V., Graves, D., & Greene, M. (2007). The uniform post-acute assessment tool: systematically evaluating the quality of measurement evidence. *Archives of Physical Medicine and Rehabilitation, 88*, 11, 1505–1512.

May, W. W. (1998). A field application of the ASAM Placement Criteria in a 12-step model of treatment for chemical dependency. *Journal of Addictive Diseases, 17*, 2, 77–91.

McKay, J. R., Cacciola, J. S., McLellan, A. T., Alterman, A. I., & Wirtz, P. W. (1997). An initial evaluation of the psychosocial dimensions of the American Society of Addiction Medicine criteria for inpatient vs. intensive outpatient substance abuse rehabilitation. *Journal of Studies on Alcohol, 58*, 5, 239–252.

Mee-Lee, D., & Shulman, G. D. (2009). The ASAM Placement Criteria and matching patients to treatment. In R. K. Ries, S. Miller, D. A. Fiellin, R. Saitz. (Eds.). *Principles of Addiction Medicine.* (4th ed., pp. 387–399). Philadelphia, PA: Lippincott Williams & Wilkins.

Mee-Lee, D. (2001). Treatment planning for dual disorders. *Psychiatric Rehabilitation Skills, 5*, 1, 52–79.

Mee-Lee, D., Shulman, G. D., Fishman, M., Gastfreid, D. R., & Griffith, J. H. (2001). *ASAM patient placement criteria for the treatment of substance related disorders, second edition-revised (ASAM PPC-2R).* Chevy Chase, MD: American Society of Addiction Medicine.

Miller, W. R., & Rollnick, S. (2002). *Motivational interviewing: preparing people for change.* New York, NY: Guilford Press.

Minkoff, K., Zweben, J., Rosenthal, R., & Ries, R. (2003). Development of service intensity criteria and program categories for individuals with co-occurring disorders. *Journal of Addict Diseases, 22*(Suppl.1), 113–129.

National Institute on Drug Abuse. (1999). *Principles of drug addiction treatment: A research-based guide* (NIH Publication # 99-4180). Rockville, MD: NIDA, National Institutes of Health.

Penberthy, J. K., Ait-Daoud, N., Breton, M., Kovatchev, B., DiClemente, C. C., & Johnson, B. A. (2007). Evaluating readiness and treatment seeking effects in a pharmacotherapy trial for alcohol dependence. *Alcoholism, Clinical and Experimental Research, 31*, 9, 1538–1544.

Peterson, A. M. (2007). Improving adherence in patients with alcohol dependence: A new role for pharmacists. *American Journal of Health System Pharmacy, 64*(5 Suppl 3), S23–29.

Rawson, R. A., & Ling, W. (n.d.). American Society of Addiction Medicine patient placement criteria for the treatment of psychoactive substance use disorders: An analysis. Unpublished paper prepared for the California Office of Alcohol and Drug Programs.

Shea, C. W. (2008). From the neurobiologic basis of alcohol dependency to pharmacologic treatment strategies: Bridging the knowledge gap. *The Southern Medical Journal, 101*, 2, 179–185.

Soyka, M., Kranzler, H. R., Berglund, M., Gorelick, D., Hesselbrock, V., Johnson, B. A., et al. (2008). World Federation of Societies of Biological Psychiatry (WFSBP) guidelines for biological treatment of substance use and related disorders, Part 1: Alcoholism. *The World Journal of Biological Psychiatry, 9*, 1, 6–23.

Swift, R. (2007). Emerging approaches to managing alcohol dependence. *American Journal of Health System Pharmacy, 64*(5 Suppl 3), S12–22.

Zweben, A., Pettinati, H. M., Weiss, R. D., Youngblood, M., Cox, C. E., Mattson, M. E., et al. (2008). Relationship between medication adherence and treatment outcomes: The COMBINE study. *Alcoholism, Clinical Experimental Research, 32*(9), 1661–1669.

CHAPTER 3

Strategies for Managing Alcohol Withdrawal

Physical addiction to alcohol is a later stage development in alcohol dependence. For patients who require detoxification or who present in withdrawal, an accurate assessment is essential to appropriate management of withdrawal, which can be life-threatening.

The patient's risk rating can be determined by completing two types of assessment: a baseline assessment of the patient's status at the initial presentation and follow-up assessments of the patient's response to treatment.

ASSESSING THE RISK OF WITHDRAWAL

Intoxication

Clinical Presentation

As blood alcohol concentration rises, so too does the clinical effect on the individual. At a blood alcohol concentration (BAC) between 20 mg% (0.02 BAC) and 99 mg% (0.099 BAC), loss of muscular coordination begins. Changes in mood, personality, and behavior accompany these blood alcohol levels. As the blood alcohol level rises to the range of l00 mg% (0.100 BAC) to 199 mg% (0.199 BAC), neurologic impairment occurs, accompanied by prolonged reaction time, ataxia, poor coordination, and mental impairment.

At a blood alcohol level of 200 mg% (0.200 BAC) to 299 mg% (0.299 BAC), very obvious intoxication is present, except in individuals with marked tolerance. Nausea and vomiting, as well as marked ataxia, may occur. As the level rises to 300 mg% (0.300 BAC) to 399 mg% (0.399 BAC), hypothermia may occur, along with severe dysarthria and amnesia, with Stage I anesthesia.

At blood alcohol levels between 400 mg% (0.400 BAC) and 799 mg% (0.799 BAC), the onset of alcoholic coma occurs. The precise level at which this occurs depends on tolerance; some persons experience coma at levels of 400 mg%, while others do not experience it until the level approaches 600 mg%.

Serum levels of alcohol between 600 mg% (0.600 BAC) and 800 mg% (0.800 BAC) often are fatal. Progressive obtundation develops, accompanied by reductions in respiration, blood pressure, and body temperature. The patient may develop urinary incontinence or retention, while reflexes are markedly decreased or absent. Death may occur from the loss of airway protective reflexes (with subsequent airway obstruction by the flaccid tongue), from pulmonary aspiration of gastric contents, or from respiratory arrest arising from profound central nervous system (CNS) depression (Mayo-Smith, 2003).

WITHDRAWAL

Clinical Presentation

The clinical manifestations of alcohol withdrawal begin 6 to 24 hours after the last drink, sometimes emerging even before the blood alcohol level has returned to zero. Early withdrawal signs and symptoms include anxiety, sleep disturbances, vivid dreams, anorexia, nausea, and headache. Physical signs include tachycardia, elevation of blood pressure, hyperactive reflexes, sweating, and hyperthermia. A tremor, best brought out by extension of the hands or tongue, may appear; this tremor has a rate of 6 to 8 cycles per second and appears on electromyography to be an exaggeration of normal physiologic tremor.

Alcohol withdrawal hallucinosis tends to occur within 12 hours of cessation. Alcohol withdrawal seizures can occur at various times, but most occur within 48 hours of cessation. Alcohol withdrawal delirium, or delirium tremens, typically begins 48 to 72 hours after the last drink and is preceded by the typical signs and symptoms of early withdrawal, although these may be masked or delayed by other illnesses or medications.

Signs of sympathetic hyperactivity (such as tachycardia, hypertension, fever, and diaphoresis) often are profound and are hallmarks of alcohol withdrawal delirium. The mortality rate is thought to be 1% to 5% and increases with delayed diagnosis, inadequate treatment, and concurrent medical conditions.

Baseline Assessment

Contrary to the expectation of many practitioners, alcoholic patients often minimize their current symptoms. For example, obtaining a previous history of withdrawal symptoms is vital, yet patients may not disclose past episodes of hallucinations or delirium tremens because of embarrassment or amnesia. When available, information from third parties can be very helpful.

It also is important to know whether the patient is also addicted to benzodiazepines or opioids, whether he or she is using other drugs, and whether the patient has other acute or chronic medical conditions and how severe they are. It is important for practitioners to specifically ask about nonmedical use of medications, even if prescribed, because such use can significantly affect the severity of alcohol withdrawal.

Biological Elements

Biological elements include:

- Presenting blood alcohol level;
- Duration of the current drinking episode;
- Whether alcohol is consumed daily and, if so, whether use typically begins in the morning or later in the day (afternoon or evening);
- The presence or absence of current withdrawal symptoms and, if present, whether they are intensifying or subsiding; and
- The number of hours since the last drink.

TABLE 3-1

Clinical Institute Withdrawal Assessment for Alcohol, Revised (CIWA-Ar)

The CIWA-Ar scale can measure 10 symptoms. Scores of less than 8 to 10 indicate minimal to mild withdrawal. Scores of 8 to 15 indicate moderate withdrawal (marked autonomic arousal), and scores of 15 or more indicate severe withdrawal. The maximum score is 67. The assessment requires 2 minutes to perform (Sullivan et al., 1989). CIWA-Ar categories, with the range of scores in each category, are as follows:

Agitation	(0–7)
Anxiety	(0–7)
Auditory disturbances	(0–7)
Clouding of Sensorium	(0–4)
Headache	(0–7)
Nausea/Vomiting	(0–7)
Paroxysmal Sweats	(0–7)
Tactile disturbances	(0–7)
Tremor	(0–7)
Visual disturbances	(0–7)

A study of the revised version of the CIWA predicted that those with a score of >15 were at increased risk for severe alcohol withdrawal (relative risk [RR] 3.72; 95% confidence interval [CI] 2.85–4.85); the higher the score, the greater the risk. Some patients (6.4%) still suffered complications, despite low scores, if left untreated (Foy et al., 1988).

At times, patients will not be honest about the number of hours that have elapsed since the last drink, particularly if they are embarrassed about having used alcohol shortly before the interview. A breath analyzer is useful in clarifying this issue (as when the reading is positive but the patient denies having had a drink in the preceding 24 hours). On the other hand, because of high tolerance, the patient may have stopped drinking the evening before and still present at a morning interview with a level in excess of 0.10 mg%.

The Clinical Institute Withdrawal Assessment for Alcohol, Revised (CIWA-Ar Scale; see Table 3-1) is a useful tool for monitoring a patient's progress in treatment, but less so for determining the initial level of care. The CIWA-Ar looks at nausea and vomiting; tremor or sweats; tactile, auditory, and visual disturbances; anxiety and agitation; headache; and disorientation or clouding of the sensorium. While CIWA-Ar scores are widely used and may be somewhat helpful as a general guide to the overall severity of withdrawal symptoms, they should not be regarded as comprehensive, because they do not reflect vital signs and do not take into account the relative weight of particular features of withdrawal, such as tremulousness, confusion, and psychosis. The presence of particular clinical signs and symptoms (as outlined in this text) should be taken as "red flags" and used as a more important guide to level of care decisions. CIWA-Ar scores are more useful as a *monitoring tool* to track the changing severity of withdrawal for a particular patient over time in response to treatment.

Psychological Elements

Psychological elements include the extent to which the patient is likely to cooperate with the detoxification process. This is determined by the patient's level of cooperation during past treatment attempts; his or her attitude toward their alcohol dependence, personality type, and approach to treatment of any medical condition; and intelligence and cognitive status.

Another consideration is the presence or absence of co-occurring Axis I psychiatric disorders and, if present, whether they are being treated and whether they are stable.

Social Elements

These include the patient's living environment and the nature of his or her relationships with family members and close friends. Of particular relevance are how understanding family and friends are about the patient's alcohol problems and how supportive they are of his or her recovery.

The attitudes and culture of the patient's broader social environment toward alcohol use disorders also are important influences.

Follow-up Assessments

The alcohol withdrawal syndrome usually evolves in a predictable pattern. Frequent reassessment is necessary to ensure safe and effective treatment. The following issues can be used as guidelines:

- Prevention of symptoms is a safer strategy than running the risk of falling behind the evolution of the withdrawal syndrome. A past history of severe withdrawal symptoms often necessitates a more aggressive medication regimen. This may involve initiating medication before the onset of significant symptoms.
- Clinical scales such as the CIWA-Ar (see Table 3-1) are helpful in assessing the patient's response to treatment.
- Anxiety and ability to sleep are the most sensitive parameters in this regard. Blood pressure and pulse, although readily measurable, tend to be overvalued and are not as useful as the patient's level of anxiety and ability to sleep in making medication decisions. For some patients, tremor can be persistent and should not be used as a parameter to determine medication after the first 36 to 48 hours. Serial breath analysis for alcohol is useful to document the steady decline in BAC and to detect any covert drinking.
- Access to all levels of care should be available from the beginning of treatment so that support can be slowly reduced as the patient progresses or intensified if the response to treatment is not sufficient.

MANAGEMENT OF ALCOHOL WITHDRAWAL

Benzodiazepines for Alcohol Withdrawal

The medical literature on the pharmacologic management of alcohol withdrawal has been comprehensively reviewed as part of the American Society of Addiction Medicine's efforts to develop evidence-based clinical practice guidelines. The evidence reviewed supported the conclusion that the cornerstone of pharmacologic management of alcohol withdrawal is the use of benzodiazepines (Mayo-Smith, 1997).

Benzodiazepines are pharmacologically cross-tolerant with alcohol and have the similar effect of enhancing GABA-induced sedation.

Formulations
Multiple oral and parenteral formulations are available.

Status
Most benzodiazepines have been placed in Schedule IV of the Federal Controlled Substances Act.

Mechanism of Action
A specific benzodiazepine receptor site has been identified on the GABA receptor complex. It is believed that the provision of benzodiazepines alleviates the acute deficiency of GABA neurotransmitter activity that occurs with sudden cessation of alcohol intake.

Safety
Benzodiazepines have a well documented margin of safety for short-term use, with a low risk of respiratory depression when taken orally, except when mixed with alcohol. They do have a potential for abuse, which increases with alcohol dependence, but is less than that of many nonbenzodiazepine sedative-hypnotics.

Evidence of Effectiveness
Well designed studies consistently have shown that benzodiazepines are more effective than placebo in reducing the signs and symptoms of withdrawal. Excellent summaries of these protocols for basic detoxification (Mayo-Smith, 1997) and for withdrawal delirium (Mayo-Smith et al., 2004) are available. In addition, metaanalysis of prospective placebo controlled trials of benzodiazepines for patients admitted with symptomatic withdrawal shows a highly significant reduction in seizures, with a risk reduction of 7.7 seizures per 100 patients treated, as well as in delirium, with a risk reduction of 4.9 cases of delirium per 100 patients treated (Kasser, Mayo-Smith et al., 1998).

Selection of a Specific Benzodiazepine
Most addiction specialists prefer to use the long-acting, low potency chlordiazepoxide or diazepam for routine detoxification. These medications are more calming, are easier to taper, are not associated with rebound withdrawal symptoms, and may be more effective in preventing seizures. Because of its lipophilic properties, diazepam enters the brain more rapidly (but this is not clinically significant) and is offset by its tendency to create euphoria, which is undesirable with addicted patients.

Despite the advantages of these two agents, nonspecialists tend to use the shorter acting, high potency lorazepam. Because lorazepam is well absorbed intramuscularly (IM), it is preferable for the small subset of patients who are unable to tolerate oral formulations. Because it is not metabolized in the liver, it also is useful for patients with severely compromised hepatic function (i.e., dysfunction that has progressed beyond simple elevation of liver function enzymes). Oxazepam, which lacks active hepatic metabolites, would be a less addictive alternative to lorazepam for patients with severely compromised liver function, as well as for elderly patients who metabolize benzodiazepines more slowly, or for patients with a history of benzodiazepine abuse, because it has lower abuse liability than other benzodiazepines.

Cautions and Contraindications

The main complication of therapy with intravenous (IV) diazepam is respiratory depression. Accordingly, providers should have equipment and personnel immediately available to provide respiratory support if needed. One advantage of diazepam is that its peak onset occurs within 5 minutes of IV administration. This allows the provider to deliver repeat boluses and titrate sedation quickly without fear of a delayed appearance of over-sedation.

Massive doses of benzodiazepines may be needed to control the agitation of patients experiencing delirium tremens, with hundreds and even thousands of milligrams of diazepam or its equivalent used over the course of treatment. The practitioner should not hesitate to use whatever amounts are needed to control the agitation.

Use in Pregnancy

Benzodiazepines are classified in FDA pregnancy Category C (adverse effects on the fetus in animal studies, but no human trials). Studies of benzodiazepine teratogenicity in humans have had conflicting results. In most cases, the risks of uncontrolled withdrawal seizures, agitation, and delirium outweigh the risks of benzodiazepine use for both the woman and her fetus. To avoid fetal or neonatal toxicity, doses of all medications should be kept as low as possible while keeping the patient stable. If significant toxicity occurs, flumazenil can be administered to the neonate. The newborn should be monitored carefully for recurring signs of toxicity, since flumazenil has a short half-life and repeat doses often are required.

Dose and Duration of Therapy

In the majority of studies examining the effectiveness of various medications for withdrawal, the medications were given in fixed amounts at scheduled times (such as chlordiazepoxide 50 mg every 6 hours) for periods of 5 to 7 days. An alternative to such a fixed schedule is known as symptom-triggered therapy. In this approach, the patient is monitored through use of a structured assessment scale and given medication only when symptoms cross a specified threshold of severity. Well-designed studies have demonstrated that this approach is as effective as fixed-dose therapy, but leads to the administration of significantly less medication and a significantly shorter duration of treatment.

Symptom-triggered therapy also facilitates the delivery of large amounts of medication quickly to patients who evidence rapidly escalating withdrawal and thus reduces the risk of undertreatment that may arise with the use of fixed doses.

For programs specializing in the management of addiction, use of a symptom-triggered approach in combination with a severity scale offers significant advantages. However, there may be situations in which the provision of fixed doses remains appropriate. For example, when a patient is admitted to a general medical or surgical unit, the nursing staff may not have the training or experience to implement the regular use of scales for patient monitoring. In certain nonhospital settings, where nursing and medical resources are limited, it may be more efficient to implement fixed-dose protocols for the majority of patients, with individualization outside of the protocol as needed. In certain patients, such as those with severe coronary artery disease, the clinician may wish to avoid symptom-triggered approaches in order to prevent the development of even minor symptoms of withdrawal.

Because a history of past withdrawal seizures is a risk factor for seizures during future withdrawal episodes, and because withdrawal seizures usually occur early in the course of withdrawal, some practitioners administer fixed doses to patients with a history of withdrawal seizures, using higher doses than they might otherwise give if using a symptom-triggered approach.

Whenever fixed doses are given, it is very important that allowances be made to provide additional medication if the fixed dose should prove inadequate to control symptoms. Treatment should allow for a degree of individualization so that patients can receive large amounts of medication rapidly if needed.

In all cases, benzodiazepines should be administered by a route that has been shown to have reliable absorption. Because of the poor IM absorption of most benzodiazepines, they should be administered orally or, when necessary, intravenously.

Adjunctive Medications for Alcohol Withdrawal

In the management of an agitated patient, benzodiazepines can be supplemented with neuroleptic agents such as haloperidol. As has been discussed, such agents should not be used alone. Also, neuroleptic agents with less effect on seizure threshold (such as haloperidol) should be used.

In patients whose withdrawal is not readily controlled with oral benzodiazepines and who are beginning to demonstrate signs of agitation, IM administration of a combination of lorazepam and a neuroleptic such as haloperidol often is effective in calming the patient, thus avoiding the need to use IV administration. However, progressive agitation generally should be considered a sign of undertreated withdrawal, calling for increased doses of benzodiazepines.

Alcohol can impair gluconeogenesis, with an increased risk of hypoglycemia, and chronic alcoholism places the individual at increased risk of thiamine deficiency. It also is important to assess whether the patient has ingested other drugs in addition to alcohol, as these may further suppress the central nervous system and alter the approach to treatment (Mayo-Smith, 2003).

Carbamazepine sometimes is used as an adjunctive agent in the management of patients who have a history of recurrent withdrawal seizures, prominent mood lability during withdrawal, or who are experiencing concurrent benzodiazepine withdrawal.

Although not frequently seen today, alcoholic patients are at risk for thiamine deficiency, which may lead to Wernicke's disease and the Wernicke-Korsakoff syndrome. Wernicke's disease is an illness of acute onset characterized by the triad of mental disturbance, paralysis of eye movements, and ataxia. The ocular abnormality usually is weakness or paralysis of abduction (sixth nerve palsy), which invariably is bilateral, although rarely symmetric. It is accompanied by diplopia, strabismus, and nystagmus. The ataxia primarily affects gait and stance. Mental status changes typically involve delirium with a global confusional-apathetic state but, in some patients, a disproportionate disorder of retentive memory is apparent.

Wernicke's disease is a neurologic emergency that should be treated by the immediate parenteral administration of thiamine, with a dose of 50 mg IV and 50 mg IM. Delay in provision of thiamine increases the risk of permanent memory damage. The provision of IV glucose solutions may exhaust a patient's reserve of B vitamins, acutely precipitating Wernicke's disease. Therefore, IV glucose always should be accompanied by the administration of thiamine in the alcoholic patient. Ocular palsies may respond within hours, while the gait and cognitive problems of Wernicke's disease improve more slowly.

As the apathy, drowsiness, and confusion recede, the patient may be left with a sometimes permanent defect in retentive memory and learning known as Korsakoff's psychosis. To reduce the risk of these sequelae, all patients presenting with alcohol withdrawal should receive 50 to 100 mg of thiamine at the time of presentation, followed by oral supplementation for several weeks. Patients with symptoms of Wernicke's disease, those who are to receive glucose-containing IV solutions, and those at high risk of malnutrition should receive their initial dose parenterally.

Alternative Medications for Detoxification

Studies have indicated that some nonbenzodiazepine sedative-hypnotics also are effective in reducing the signs and symptoms of withdrawal. For example, phenobarbital—a long-acting barbiturate—still is used by some programs because it is long-acting, has well documented anticonvulsant activity, is inexpensive, and has comparatively low abuse liability.

Although phenobarbital sometimes has been recommended as a replacement for benzodiazepines in alcohol detoxification during pregnancy, it confers no significant advantage. Like benzodiazepines, it can cause fetal or neonatal toxicity. In addition, most studies suggest phenobarbital is a weak teratogen, causing an increase in minor craniofacial anomalies and possibly an increase in nonspecific major anomalies. As with phenobarbital, there is no evidence that chloral hydrate is safer during pregnancy than benzodiazepines. Limited data suggest that it may have nonspecific teratogenic effects, and that it may have more side effects in the newborn than benzodiazepines.

Beta-adrenergic blocking agents, such as atenolol and propranolol, as well as centrally acting alpha-adrenergic agonists, such as clonidine, also are effective in ameliorating symptoms in patients with mild to moderate withdrawal, primarily by reducing the autonomic nervous system manifestations of withdrawal. However, these agents do not have known anticonvulsant activity and are unlikely to reduce seizures or delirium. Beta-blockers pose a particular problem in this regard because delirium is a known, albeit rare, side effect of these drugs. In addition, there is concern that selective reduction in certain manifestations of withdrawal may mask the development of other significant withdrawal symptoms and make it difficult to utilize withdrawal scales to guide therapy.

The beta-adrenergic blocking agents propranolol and atenolol have been relatively well studied during pregnancy and have not been associated with adverse effects. Propranolol can have a greater effect on heart rate during pregnancy than in the nonpregnant state, so heart rate should be closely monitored. Atenolol has a theoretical advantage over propranolol because it is a selective beta-1 receptor blocker, so it does not block beta-2 uterine receptors to increase myometrial tone. In sum, untreated withdrawal symptoms in pregnancy clearly pose a greater risk than treatment with atenolol or propranolol.

Anticonvulsants such as carbamazepine and gabapentin have been the subject of studies of their effectiveness as alternative medications for mild to moderate withdrawal. These agents are especially useful in ambulatory settings because they offer lower sedating properties and almost no risk of abuse. Carbamazepine has been widely used for alcohol withdrawal in Europe, where it has been shown to equal benzodiazepines in efficacy for patients with mild to moderate withdrawal. It is without significant toxicity when used in 7-day protocols for alcohol withdrawal and is associated with less psychiatric distress and a more rapid return to work.

Carbamazepine does not potentiate the CNS and respiratory depression caused by alcohol, does not cause cognitive impairment (an important side effect of larger doses of benzodiazepines), and has no abuse potential. During pregnancy, its use poses a number of risks. During the first trimester, it is weakly teratogenic, increasing the risk of minor congenital anomalies, neural tube defects, and possibly developmental delay. Given later in pregnancy, in rare instances it can increase the risk of neonatal hemorrhage by lowering vitamin K-dependent coagulation factors or cause transient neonatal hepatic dysfunction.

Neuroleptic agents demonstrate some effectiveness in reducing the signs and symptoms of withdrawal and, for a period of time, were used extensively for that purpose. However, these agents are less effective than benzodiazepines in preventing delirium and actually can lead to an increase in the rate of seizures. Neuroleptic agents are widely used to calm agitated patients and are useful for this purpose in the setting of alcohol withdrawal as well. They should not be used alone, but always concurrently with a benzodiazepine; moreover, neuroleptic agents with less effect on the seizure threshold, such as haloperidol, should be selected.

An agent whose use for the management of alcohol withdrawal still is encountered occasionally is alcohol itself. Case series describing oral or IV alcohol for the prevention or treatment of withdrawal symptoms have been published, but no controlled trials evaluating the safety or relative efficacy of this approach—either compared to placebo or to benzodiazepines—have been performed. IV alcohol infusions require close monitoring because of the potential toxicity of alcohol. As a pharmacologic agent, ethyl alcohol has numerous adverse effects, including its well known hepatic, gastrointestinal, pancreatic, and neurologic toxicities. Given the proven efficacy and safety of benzodiazepines, the use of alcohol for detoxification is discouraged by addiction specialists.

Clinical Recommendation

Based on the weight of evidence for their effectiveness, benzodiazepines are recommended as the pharmacotherapies of choice in the management of acute alcohol withdrawal.

Nonpharmacologic Therapies for Alcohol Withdrawal

Supportive nonpharmacologic care is an important and useful element in the management of all patients undergoing withdrawal. Simple interventions such as reassurance, reality orientation, monitoring of signs and symptoms of withdrawal, and general nursing care are effective. In controlled trials, they were sufficient to manage 85% of emergency room patients and 60% of inpatients (Sellers, Naranjo, & Peachey, 1981). However, it is important to understand that these measures do not prevent the development of major complications such as seizures and are not adequate by themselves to manage the patient with severe withdrawal or delirium, in which case pharmacologic intervention is required.

In all cases of withdrawal, supportive and comforting nonpharmacologic interventions should be considered important adjuncts to pharmacologic treatments. In cases of mild withdrawal, such nonpharmacologic approaches may be the mainstay of treatment, so long as adequate provision is made for trained personnel to monitor the patient for potential worsening of symptoms or the development of unexpectedly severe withdrawal symptoms.

The use of "social detoxification" always should include provision for back-up medical evaluation and treatment (i.e., so-called "rescue protocols") for the introduction of pharmacologic therapies as needed. Certain symptoms are particularly important indicators of the presence of moderate to severe withdrawal and are predictive of the need for pharmacologic therapies. These include tremor, elevation of heart rate and blood pressure, sensory disturbance, changes in level of consciousness, disorientation, or confusion.

For a brief review of selected nonpharmacologic therapies, see Appendix B.

REFERENCES

American Psychiatric Association. (2000). *Diagnostic and statistical manual of mental disorders, fourth edition, text revision (DSM-IV-TR)*. Washington, DC: American Psychiatric Press.

Center for Substance Abuse Treatment. (2005). *Substance abuse treatment for persons with co-Occurring disorders. Treatment improvement protocol (TIP) Series 42*. (DHHS Publication No. (SMA) 05-3992.) Rockville, MD: Substance Abuse and Mental Health Services Administration.

Foy, A., March, S., & Drinkwater, V. (1988). Use of an objective clinical scale in the assessment and management of alcohol withdrawal in a large general hospital. *Alcoholism: Clinical and Experimental Research, 12*, 360–364.

Hartsell, Z., Drost, J., Wilkens, J. A., & Budavari, A. I. (2007). Managing alcohol withdrawal in hospitalized patients. *Journal of the American Academy of Addiction Psychiatry, 20*, 9, 20–25.

Hilton, T. (2007). Pharmacological issues in the management of people with mental illness and problems with alcohol and illicit drug misuse. *Criminal Behavior and Mental Health, 17*, 4, 215–224.

Kasser, C., Mayo-Smith, M., et al. (1998). *Management of alcohol withdrawal delirium (clinical practice guideline)*. Chevy Chase, MD: American Society of Addiction Medicine.

Mayo-Smith, M. F. (1997). Pharmacological management of alcohol withdrawal: A meta-analysis and evidence-based practice guideline. *Journal of the American Medical Association, 278*, 2, 144–151.

Mayo-Smith, M. F. (2003). Management of alcohol withdrawal. In: A. W. Graham, T. K. Schultz, M. F. Mayo-Smith, R. K. Ries, & B. B. Wilford (Eds.), *Principles of addiction medicine* (3rd ed.). Chevy Chase, MD: American Society of Addiction Medicine. Erratum (dosage error in text) in Oct. 11, *164*, 18, 2068.

Mayo-Smith, M. F., Beecher, L. H., Fischer, T. L., Gorelick, D. A., Guillaume, J. L., Hill, A., et al., for the Working Group on the Management of Alcohol Withdrawal Delirium, Practice Guidelines Committee, American Society of Addiction Medicine. (2004). Management of alcohol withdrawal delirium. An evidence-based practice guideline. *Archives of Internal Medicine, 164*, 13, 1405–1412.

McKeon, A., Frye, N. A., & Delanty, N. (2008). The alcohol withdrawal syndrome. *Journal of Neurolpgy, Neurosurgery, and Psychiatry, 79*, 854–862.

Miller, L, (2003). Detoxification of the addicted woman in pregnancy. In A. W. Graham, T. K. Schultz, M. F. Mayo-Smith, R. K. Ries, & B. B. Wilford (Eds.). *Principles of addiction medicine* (3rd ed.). Chevy Chase, MD: American Society of Addiction Medicine.

Sellers, E. M., Naranjo, C. A., & Peachey, J. E. (1981). Drug therapy: drugs to decrease alcohol consumption. *New England Journal of Medicine, 305*, 21, 1255–1262.

Sullivan, J. T., Sykora, K., Schneiderman, J., Naranjo C. A., & Sellers, E. M. (1989). Assessment of alcohol withdrawal: The revised Clinical Institute Withdrawal Instrument for Alcohol Scale (CIWA-Ar). *British Journal of Addiction,* 84, 1353–1357.

Uzbay, I. T. (2008). Serotonergic anti-depressants and ethanol withdrawal syndrome: A review. *Alcohol and Alcoholism, 43*, 1, 15–24.

Weaver, M. F. (2003). Management of the addicted woman in pregnancy. In A. W. Graham, T. K. Schultz, M. F. Mayo-Smith, R. K. Ries, & B. B. Wilford (Eds.), *Principles of addiction medicine* (3rd ed.). Chevy Chase, MD: American Society of Addiction Medicine.

Ziegler, P. P. (2007). Alcohol use and anxiety. *American Journal of Psychiatry,* 164, 8, 1270.

CHAPTER 4

Placement Criteria for Managing Alcohol Withdrawal

TREATMENT LEVELS WITHIN DIMENSION 1

Dimension 1, Acute Intoxication and/or Withdrawal Potential, is the first of the six primary assessment areas to be evaluated in making treatment and placement decisions. The range of clinical severity seen in this dimension has given rise to multiple levels of service intensity in the management of detoxification.

In this context, detoxification refers not only to the attenuation of the physiologic and psychologic features of withdrawal syndromes, but also to the process of interrupting the momentum of compulsive use in persons diagnosed with substance *dependence*. Because of the force of this momentum and the inherent difficulties in overcoming it even when there is no clear withdrawal syndrome, this phase of treatment frequently requires a greater intensity of services initially to establish treatment engagement and patient role induction. This is, of course, critical to the course of treatment, because it is not possible to engage a patient in treatment while that patient is caught up in a cycle of frequent intoxication and withdrawal.

Detoxification is best viewed as an opportunity to introduce the patient to the recovery process. In contrast, approaching detoxification as an isolated procedure can perpetuate a "revolving door" cycle of stagnant chronicity. Patients need to understand that detoxification is just the first step in their treatment. The detoxification process always should be embedded in a program of rehabilitation rather than being addressed as a discrete medical procedure. Modern detoxification protocols are so effective that patients usually can participate in group and individual therapy from the first day of treatment.

Level I-D: Ambulatory Detoxification Without Extended On-site Monitoring

Level I-D detoxification is an organized outpatient service, which may be delivered in an office setting, health care or addiction treatment facility, or in a patient's home by trained clinicians who provide medically supervised evaluation, detoxification, and referral services according to a predetermined schedule. Such services are provided in regularly scheduled sessions.

Level I-D services should be delivered under a defined set of policies and procedures or clinical protocols. Outpatient detoxification services should be designed to treat the patient's level of clinical severity and to achieve safe and comfortable withdrawal from mood-altering drugs (including alcohol), as well as to facilitate the patient's transition into ongoing treatment and recovery.

Level II-D: Ambulatory Detoxification With Extended On-site Monitoring

Level II-D detoxification is an organized outpatient service, which may be delivered in an office setting or health care or addiction treatment facility by trained clinicians who provide medically supervised evaluation, detoxification, and referral services. Level II-D services are provided in regularly scheduled sessions. They are delivered under a defined set of policies and procedures or clinical protocols. Outpatient services are designed to treat the patient's level of clinical severity and to achieve safe and comfortable withdrawal from mood-altering drugs (including alcohol), as well as to facilitate the patient's entry into ongoing treatment and recovery.

Essential to this level of care is the availability of appropriately credentialed and licensed nurses (such as registered nurses or licensed practical nurses), who monitor patients over a period of several hours each day of service.

Level III-D: Residential/Inpatient Detoxification

Criteria are provided for two types of Level III detoxification programs: Level III.2-D (Clinically Managed Residential Detoxification) and Level III.7-D (Medically Monitored Inpatient Detoxification). The "residential" level of care has, in the past, been synonymous with rehabilitation services, whereas detoxification services and the "inpatient" level of care have been synonymous with acute inpatient hospital care. With the increased availability and utilization of Medically Monitored Inpatient Detoxification services, the terms "residential" and "inpatient" are being used more broadly to contrast ambulatory ("outpatient") detoxification with nonambulatory ("residential" or "inpatient") detoxification services. The difference between these two levels of detoxification is the intensity of clinical services, particularly as demonstrated by the degree of involvement of medical and nursing professionals.

Level III.2-D, Clinically Managed Residential Detoxification (sometimes referred to as "social setting detoxification"), is an organized service that may be delivered by appropriately trained staff who provide 24-hour supervision, observation, and support for patients who are intoxicated or experiencing withdrawal. Clinically managed residential detoxification is characterized by its emphasis on peer and social support.

Level III.2-D programs care for patients whose intoxication/withdrawal signs and symptoms are so severe as to require 24-hour structure and support, but who do not need the full resources of a Level III.7-D medically monitored inpatient detoxification service. In some clinically managed residential detoxification programs, staff supervise patients as they self-administer medications for the management of withdrawal. All programs at this level rely on established clinical protocols to identify patients who are in need of medical services beyond the capacity of the facility, and they are prepared to transfer such patients to more appropriate levels of care.

Level III.7-D, Medically Monitored Inpatient Detoxification, is an organized service delivered by medical and nursing professionals, which provides for 24-hour medically supervised evaluation and withdrawal management in a permanent facility with inpatient beds. Services are delivered under a defined set of physician-approved policies and physician-monitored procedures or clinical protocols. This level provides care to patients whose withdrawal signs and symptoms are so severe as to require 24-hour inpatient care. Services sometimes are provided in coordination with Level IV-D services (as a "step-down" service) in a specialty unit of an acute care general or psychiatric hospital, or as part of a Level III. 7-Medically Monitored Intensive Inpatient Treatment program. Twenty-four hour observation, monitoring, and treatment are available; however, the full resources of an acute care general hospital or a medically managed intensive inpatient treatment program are not necessary.

Level IV-D: Medically Managed Intensive Inpatient Detoxification

Level IV-D detoxification is an organized service delivered by medical and nursing professionals, who provide 24-hour medically directed evaluation and withdrawal management in an acute care inpatient setting. Services are delivered under a defined set of physician-approved policies and physician-managed procedures or medical protocols.

Level IV-D provides care to patients whose withdrawal signs and symptoms are so severe as to require primary medical and nursing care services. Twenty-four hour observation, monitoring, and treatment are available. Although Level IV-D is specifically designed for acute medical detoxification, as with all the levels of detoxification, it also is important to assess the patient and develop a care plan for any treatment priorities identified in Dimensions 2 through 6.

RISK ASSESSMENT MATRIX FOR DIMENSION 1

In each assessment dimension (which correspond to Dimensions 1 to 6 of the ASAM Patient Placement Criteria), the Risk Rating (first column of the Matrix) suggests the severity of the patient's problem in that dimension. The treatment priorities represented by the Service Needs and Interventions (second column of the Matrix) suggest the specific types of treatment services/modalities the patient requires to appropriately address his or her multidimensional service needs. The Level of Care and Setting (third column of the Matrix) suggests the intensity and resources with which those services can be effectively delivered within a range of settings and levels of care.

MATRIX FOR DIMENSION 1: WITHDRAWAL

The patient's assessed needs should be considered in each ASAM Dimension. The interaction between Dimension 1 and other Dimensions may increase or reduce assessed severity (see the discussion of Dimensional interactions in Chapter 2).

RISK RATING	SERVICE NEEDS AND INTERVENTIONS	LEVEL OF CARE AND SETTING
General Considerations Considerations and services that are common to all risk levels are described here. The sections that follow identify issues and services that have particular relevance to or urgency for patients with specific Risk Ratings.	**Service Needs** All patients who receive detoxification treatment should be offered immediate access to an addiction counseling program. Patients should be very strongly encouraged to immediately and simultaneously engage in, or transition to, ongoing continuing care to support relapse prevention. Education should be offered to help the patient understand the relative advantages and disadvantages of various antiaddiction medications (such as disulfiram, naltrexone, acamprosate, and sustained-release injectable naltrexone) as a potential component of relapse prevention or treatment. **Treatment Interventions** Patients may benefit from a variety of interventions (*see the discussion in Chapter 3 and Appendix B*). At lower levels of risk, patients generally benefit from a targeted selection of interventions. Patients at higher levels of risk need a broader array of coordinated interventions. If the patient's treatment has included a pharmacotherapy (such as concurrent opioid maintenance therapy [OMT] with methadone or buprenorphine), the patient should be encouraged to continue it under medical supervision. However, any pharmacotherapy should be carefully integrated into the overall treatment plan.	**Coordination of Services** Addiction treatment programs should develop referral relationships with and linkages to addiction medicine specialists who are experienced in evaluating patients and using pharmacotherapies to manage withdrawal and prevent relapse. Such services should be available as a routine component of care. When withdrawal management and addiction treatment services are delivered by separate providers, coordination is vital. **Staffing** Addiction counselors involved in the care of patients being withdrawn from alcohol should be aware of the goals of pharmacotherapy and prepared to collaborate in monitoring and supporting it. Treatment programs should have mechanisms in place (such as training, supervision, etc.) to encourage and facilitate such collaboration.

(continues)

RISK RATING	SERVICE NEEDS AND INTERVENTIONS	LEVEL OF CARE AND SETTING
	Although there have been reports of dangerous interactions between buprenorphine and benzodiazepines, those reports generally involved concurrent *intravenous* buprenorphine abuse and *intravenous* benzodiazepine abuse. The prescription of benzodiazepines for alcohol detoxification concurrent with prescription of buprenorphine—either for opioid maintenance treatment or opioid detoxification—generally is safe under close clinical monitoring and supervision. The patient who is treated with an antiaddiction medication needs frequent initial monitoring, followed by ongoing medication management. This can be performed by an appropriately trained and experienced primary care physician or a specialist in addiction medicine or addiction psychiatry.	
Risk Rating = 0 (Minimal or no risk) A Risk Rating of **0** in Dimension 1 indicates that the patient is fully functioning and demonstrates good ability to tolerate and cope with the discomfort of withdrawal. **Initial Assessment** The patient with a Risk Rating of **0** evidences no observable signs or symptoms of intoxication or withdrawal, or minor signs or symptoms are resolving and the patient is fully functioning and demonstrates good ability to tolerate and cope with any withdrawal discomfort. **Concurrent OMT** If the patient is undergoing concurrent opioid maintenance therapy (OMT), the dose is well-stabilized and the patient exhibits no evidence of opioid intoxication or withdrawal.	**Service Needs** A Risk Rating of **0** in Dimension 1 indicates that no immediate intoxication monitoring or detoxification services are needed. It does not affect the overall placement decision. **Treatment Interventions** At this level of risk, there is no need to initiate new professional services specifically for problems in Dimension 1. However, the patient may be receiving (and should continue to receive) maintenance treatment with antiaddiction medications, such as those for alcohol dependence or opioid addiction (OMT), as well as continuing care counseling, and these should be continued.	**Appropriate Level of Care or Setting** For the patient with a Risk Rating of **0** in Dimension 1, the determination of level of care or setting is guided by the risk rating in other Dimensions. **Concurrent OMT** The OMT patient who is being treated in a Level I outpatient OMT program should continue at that level of care.

Risk Rating = 1 (Mild risk)

A Risk Rating of **1** in Dimension 1 indicates that the patient is experiencing mild signs and symptoms of intoxication or withdrawal, but has an adequate ability to tolerate and cope with withdrawal discomfort.

The patient's mild signs and symptoms of intoxication or withdrawal do not pose an imminent danger to self or others. The patient is also assessed as being at minimum risk of progressing to severe withdrawal.

Initial Assessment

The patient with a Risk Rating of **1** evidences mild anxiety, sweating, and insomnia, but no tremor (generally associated with a CIWA-Ar score less than 8*). In addition:

(1) The patient is not withdrawing from other substances.

(2) He or she is fully coherent and able to comprehend instructions.

(3) The patient has no more than mild active medical problems, or any that exist (such as hypertension, diabetes, or hepatitis) are stable.

(4) There are no symptoms of a co-occurring psychiatric disorder (such as a mood, anxiety, or attention deficit disorder) or such symptoms are mild, reflecting a low level of severity, or are stable as the result of treatment.

(5) If the patient previously stopped drinking within the past year, he or she did not experience a severe withdrawal syndrome. (For example, if the patient gives a history of seizure or severe tremor within the preceding several months, it might call into question the quantity of alcohol consumed and raise concerns about the possible emergence of a more severe withdrawal syndrome than would be expected on the basis of the patient's report, raising the Risk Rating from 1 to 2).

(6) The patient has a high level of commitment to the detoxification process and is very cooperative with treatment interventions.

(7) The patient demonstrates a clear understanding of treatment instructions and has the resources to carry them out. Reliability is demonstrated by the patient's willingness to accept recommendations for treatment and responsiveness to treatment interventions.

(8) The patient has family or friends who are supportive of the detoxification process and can assist in providing transportation and a safe place to stay. Or, if such supports are absent, the patient demonstrates an ability to obtain transportation (other than driving himself or herself) and access to safe and appropriate housing.

Service Needs

A Risk Rating of **1** indicates a need for professional services, such as low-intensity intoxication monitoring or detoxification services, specifically to address problems in Dimension 1.

Immediate service needs include baseline measurement of blood alcohol level. If positive, serial measurements should be conducted until the level is zero. Urine drug testing should be conducted to detect the presence of substances other than alcohol.

Treatment Interventions

A long-acting benzodiazepine should be given. Effects should be monitored through the use of the CIWA-Ar or equivalent instrument.* Doses should be repeated, preferably daily, using a symptom-triggered or time-driven protocol, with a symptom-driven override/rescue protocol.

Anticonvulsants such as carbamazepine and gabapentin are sometimes used for mild to moderate withdrawal symptoms. For ambulatory detoxification, they offer the advantages of causing minimal sedation and not being subject to abuse.

A limited amount of medication should be prescribed or dispensed, sufficient to last until the next visit (ideally, the next day). The benzodiazepine medication should be adjusted at subsequent visits on a tapering schedule and discontinued entirely within a total treatment period of 3 to 5 days (longer in the case of additional detoxification from long-acting sedative-hypnotics).

Persistent abstinence symptoms beyond the period of acute withdrawal should not be

Appropriate Level of Care or Setting

A Risk Rating of **1** in Dimension 1 indicates the need for Level I-D ambulatory detoxification without extended onsite monitoring, if the patient has sufficient supports (such as family) to provide monitoring of symptoms.

If such supports are absent, the patient should be placed in a Level II-D detoxification program. Clinical services may be delivered in a primary care, addiction treatment, or mental health setting.

If family or other supports are not adequate or the patient meets residential criteria in other dimensions, then a Level III.2-D (clinically managed residential detoxification) program with concurrent medical services equivalent to Level I-D may be appropriate.

If the patient requires intensive mental health services (with a Risk Rating of 2 or higher in Dimension 3), low-intensity detoxification can be provided in a mental health setting, with ongoing case management to coordinate care.

Concurrent OMT

The patient on OMT requires continuation of opioid maintenance medications, such as methadone or buprenorphine, during and after detoxification, along with

(continues)

RISK RATING	SERVICE NEEDS AND INTERVENTIONS	LEVEL OF CARE AND SETTING
Concurrent OMT In a patient who is undergoing concurrent OMT, the dose of OMT medication may be inadequately stabilized and the patient may have mild symptoms of withdrawal or engage in occasional compensatory use of opiates or other drugs. **Reassessment** On reassessment after initiation of treatment, the patient with a Risk Rating of **1** evidences one of the following: (a) The patient's symptoms are improving as a result of the medical and psychosocial interventions, but sufficient residual symptoms persist to justify a continued Risk Rating of 1; ***or:*** (b) The patient's withdrawal symptoms initially were compatible with a Risk Rating of 0, but have intensified; ***or:*** (c) The patient's withdrawal symptoms initially were compatible with a Risk Rating of 2 (or higher) and have improved sufficiently in response to treatment to warrant a reduction to a Risk Rating of 1.	treated with benzodiazepines because of the danger of cross-addiction. Useful medications for ongoing symptomatic relief in the sub-acute period (days to weeks) include acamprosate and, for sleep, low doses of nonaddicting medications such as mirtazapine, trazodone, amitriptyline, ramelteon, and quetiapine The patient should be offered immediate access to, and simultaneous participation in, an addiction counseling program or other suitable psychosocial intervention (*see Appendix B*). Transportation should be arranged to return the patient to his or her home and overnight supervision.	assessment for dose adjustment, counseling services to assess and address readiness to change, relapse issues, and random urine testing. Such a patient is appropriately placed in a Level I outpatient OMT program, which may be housed in a primary care, addiction treatment, or mental health setting. During detoxification from alcohol, opioid maintenance medications should be provided either by the detoxification program or through coordination with the patient's Level I outpatient OMT program.
Risk Rating = 2 (Moderate risk) A Risk Rating of **2** in Dimension 1 indicates that the patient is experiencing moderate difficulty in tolerating and coping with the discomfort of withdrawal. Alternatively, the patient's level of intoxication or withdrawal may be severe, but it responds to support and treatment sufficiently that the patient does not pose an imminent danger to self or others. **Initial Assessment** The patient with a Risk Rating of **2** evidences one of the following: (1) The patient has moderate anxiety, sweating, and insomnia, as well as a mild tremor, indicating a moderate risk of severe withdrawal, which generally is associated with a CIWA-Ar score of 8 to 15*). He or she is not with	**Service Needs** A Risk Rating of **2** in Dimension 1 indicates the need for moderate-intensity intoxication monitoring or detoxification services. **Treatment Interventions** A long-acting benzodiazepine medication should be given. Medication effects should be monitored—preferably several times a day, in accordance with the severity and course of withdrawal symptoms—through the use of the CIWA-Ar* or an equivalent instrument. Doses should be repeated, with the capacity for dosing multiple times a day,	**Appropriate Level of Care or Setting** The patient with a Risk Rating of **2** in Dimension 1 should be placed in a Level II-D ambulatory detoxification program, with extended onsite monitoring. Such a program may be located in an addiction treatment or mental health setting. If family, transportation, or other supports are not adequate to enable the success of a Level II-D program or the patient meets residential criteria in other

drawing from a substance other than alcohol, and is fully coherent and able to comprehend instructions. In addition: a. The patient has no significant active medical problems, or any that exist (such as hypertension, diabetes, or hepatitis) are stable. Any current physical symptoms such as nausea or vomiting are no more than moderate in intensity. b. Any symptoms of a co-occurring psychiatric disorder (such as a mood, anxiety, or attention deficit disorder) are mild, reflecting a low level of severity, or are stable as the result of treatment. c. If the patient previously stopped drinking within the past year, he or she did not experience a severe withdrawal syndrome. (For example, if the patient gave a history of seizure or severe tremor within the preceding several months, it might call into question the quantity of alcohol consumed and raise concerns about the possible emergence of a more severe withdrawal syndrome than would be expected on the basis of the patient's report, raising the Risk Rating from 2 to 3). d. The patient has a high level of commitment to the detoxification process and is very cooperative. e. The patient (or his or her significant support person) demonstrates a clear understanding of treatment instructions and the resources to carry them out. Reliability is demonstrated by the patient's willingness to accept recommendations for treatment and responsiveness to treatment interventions. f. The patient has family or friends who are at least minimally supportive of the detoxification process and can assist in providing transportation and a safe place to stay. Or, if such supports are absent, the patient demonstrates an ability to obtain transportation (other than driving himself or herself) and access to safe and appropriate housing. ***or:*** (2) The patient exhibits moderate anxiety, sweating, and insomnia, but <u>no</u> tremor. He or she is not withdrawing from a substance other than alcohol, and is fully coherent and able to comprehend instructions. The patient otherwise would have had a Risk Rating of **1**, but evidences one or more of the following problems, which pose a significant impediment to detoxification at a less intensive level of care: a. The patient has moderate, active, and potentially destabilizing medical problems (either acute—such as nausea and intermittent vomiting from gastritis—or chronic, such as significant hypertension). b. Symptoms of a co-occurring psychiatric disorder (such as a mood, anxiety, or attention deficit disorder) are active, reflecting a moderate level of severity that is likely to complicate the detoxification.	using a symptom-triggered or time-driven protocol, with a symptom-driven override/rescue protocol in place. Anticonvulsants such as carbamazepine and gabapentin may be used as alternatives for mild to moderate withdrawal symptoms. For ambulatory detoxification, these medications offer the advantages of causing minimal sedation and not being subject to abuse. A limited amount of medication should be prescribed or dispensed, sufficient to last until the next visit (ideally, the next day). The benzodiazepine medication should be adjusted at subsequent visits on a tapering schedule and discontinued entirely within a total treatment period of 3 to 5 days (longer in the case of additional detoxification from long-acting sedative-hypnotics). Persistent abstinence symptoms beyond the period of acute withdrawal should not be treated with benzodiazepines because of the danger of cross-addiction. Useful medications for ongoing symptomatic relief in the subacute period (days to weeks) include acamprosate and, for sleep, low doses of nonaddicting medications such as mirtazapine, trazodone, amitriptyline, ramelteon, and quetiapine. The patient should be offered immediate access to, and simultaneous participation in, an addiction counseling program or other suitable psychosocial intervention (*see Appendix B*). Transportation to return the patient to his or her home and overnight supervision should be arranged.	Dimensions, then residential treatment supports should be added. If available, a Level III.2-D (clinically managed residential detoxification) program with concurrent medical services equivalent to Level II-D should be considered. If the patient requires partial hospitalization or more intensive mental health services (i.e., a Risk Rating of 2 or 3 or higher in Dimension 3), moderate intensity detoxification can be provided in a properly equipped mental health setting with ongoing case management to coordinate care.

(continues)

RISK RATING	SERVICE NEEDS AND INTERVENTIONS	LEVEL OF CARE AND SETTING
c. The patient's past attempts to stop drinking were marked by severe withdrawal symptoms (such as moderate to severe agitation and tremor, seizures or delirium tremens). d. The patient does not have a high level of commitment to the detoxification process and his or her level of cooperation and reliability are questionable. For example, the patient has a recent history of detoxification at less intensive levels of care that were marked by inability to complete detoxification or to enter into continuing addiction treatment, and the patient lacks sufficient skills to complete detoxification e. The patient's likelihood of imminent relapse is high. f. The patient's family or friends are not supportive of or oppose the detoxification process and will not assist in providing transportation and a safe place to stay. The patient appears unable to obtain transportation (other than driving himself or herself) and access to safe and appropriate housing.		
Concurrent OMT For the patient who is undergoing concurrent OMT, a Risk Rating of **2** is compatible with varying degrees of stability or instability of the dose, varying degrees of symptoms of opioid withdrawal, and/or concurrent illicit use of opioids. **Reassessment** On reassessment after initiation of treatment, the patient with a Risk Rating of **2** evidences one of the following: (1) The patient's symptoms are improving as a result of the medical and psychosocial interventions, but sufficient residual symptoms persist to justify a continued Risk of Rating **2**; ***or:*** (2) The patient's withdrawal symptoms initially were compatible with a Risk Rating of 1 and have intensified despite appropriate treatment; ***or:*** (3) The patient's withdrawal symptoms initially were compatible with Risk Rating 3 and have improved sufficiently in response to treatment to warrant a reduction to a Risk Rating of **2**.		**Concurrent OMT** The OMT patient who has a Risk Rating of **2** requires continuation of opioid maintenance medications, such as methadone or buprenorphine, during and after detoxification, along with assessment for dose adjustment, counseling services to assess and address readiness to change and relapse issues, and random urine testing. During detoxification from alcohol, opioid maintenance medications should be provided either by the detoxification program or through coordination with the patient's Level I outpatient OMT program.

Risk Rating = 3 (Significant risk)	**Service Needs**	**Appropriate Level of Care or Setting**
A Risk Rating of **3** in Dimension 1 indicates that the patient has significant signs and symptoms of withdrawal, or is at risk for significant but manageable withdrawal; or withdrawal is worsening despite detoxification at a less intensive level of care (e.g., because of concurrent opiate withdrawal with attendant cravings and impulsive behaviors). **Initial Assessment** The patient with a Risk Rating of **3** evidences one of the following: (1) The patient has significant anxiety and a moderate to severe tremor, which is generally associated with a CIWA-Ar score of 10 or more.* The patient also may be withdrawing from substances other than alcohol. However, he or she is fully coherent and able to comprehend instructions; ***or:*** (2) The patient has moderate anxiety, sweating, and insomnia, as well as a mild tremor, which generally is associated with a CIWA-Ar score of 8 to 15.* He or she is not withdrawing from a substance other than alcohol, and is fully coherent and able to comprehend instructions. The patient would otherwise have had a Risk Rating of 2, except that he or she evidences one or more of the following problems, which pose a significant impediment to detoxification at a less intensive level of care: a. The patient has moderate to severe active and potentially destabilizing medical problems (either acute such as nausea and intermittent vomiting from gastritis, or chronic such as severe hypertension). b. Symptoms of a co-occurring psychiatric disorder (such as a mood, anxiety, or attention deficit disorder) are moderate to severe. c. The patient's past attempts to stop drinking were marked by severe withdrawal symptoms (e.g., moderate to severe agitation and tremor, seizures, or delirium tremens). d. The patient does not have a high level of commitment to the detoxification process and his or her level of cooperation and reliability are questionable. For example, the patient has a recent history of detoxification at less intensive levels of care that were marked by inability to complete detoxification or to enter into continuing addiction treatment, and the patient lacks sufficient skills to complete detoxification. e. The patient is at significant risk of imminent relapse. f. The patient's family or friends are not supportive of or oppose the detoxification process and will not assist in providing transportation and a safe place	A Risk Rating of **3** in Dimension 1 indicates a need for moderately high-intensity intoxication monitoring or detoxification services. Nursing and medical care is essential. **Treatment Interventions** A long-acting benzodiazepine medication should be given. Medication effects should be monitored very frequently (at least several times a day, or hourly if needed in the presence of severe tremor or elevated vital signs) through the use of the CIWA-Ar* or equivalent instrument. Doses should be repeated, using a symptom-triggered or time-driven protocol, with a symptom-driven override/rescue protocol in place. If the patient is in an ambulatory setting, a limited amount of medication should be prescribed or dispensed, sufficient to last until the next day. Patients should have access to on-call medical personnel between scheduled assessments in case of worsening symptoms. The benzodiazepine medication should be adjusted at subsequent visits on a tapering schedule and discontinued entirely within a total treatment period of 3 to 5 days (longer if the patient also is being withdrawn from long-acting sedative-hypnotics). Persistent abstinence symptoms beyond the period of acute withdrawal should not be treated with benzodiazepines because of the danger of cross-addiction. Useful medications for ongoing symptomatic relief in the subacute period (days to weeks) include acamprosate and, for sleep, low doses of nonaddicting medications such as mirtazapine, trazodone, amitriptyline, ramelteon, and quetiapine. The patient should be offered immediate access to, and simultaneous participation in, a	The patient with a Risk Rating of **3** in Dimension 1 should be placed in a Level II-D (ambulatory detoxification with extended onsite monitoring) or Level III.7-D (medically monitored inpatient detoxification) program. However, Level II-D is not appropriate if certain symptoms (such as agitation or severe tremor) are persistently present at the close of the day's program service hours, because such a patient needs 24-hour medical monitoring. Level II-D also is not appropriate if assessment items 2d or 2f (see column 1 to the left) exist, unless Level II-D can be combined with a supportive living arrangement. Alternatively, the patient may be placed in a Level III.7-D medically monitored inpatient detoxification program. Such a program may be located in an addiction treatment or mental health setting. If the patient requires medically monitored or clinically-managed mental health services (with a Risk Rating of **3** or higher in Dimension 3), moderately high-intensity detoxification can be provided in a mental health setting with ongoing case management to coordinate care.

(continues)

RISK RATING	SERVICE NEEDS AND INTERVENTIONS	LEVEL OF CARE AND SETTING
to stay. The patient appears unable to obtain transportation (other than driving himself or herself) and access to safe and appropriate housing. **Concurrent OMT** For patients undergoing concurrent OMT, a Risk Rating of **3** is compatible with varying degrees of stability or instability of the dose, varying degrees of symptoms of opioid withdrawal, and/or concurrent illicit use of opioids. **Reassessment** On reassessment after initiation of treatment, the patient with a Risk Rating of **3** evidences one of the following: (1) The patient's symptoms are improving as a result of the medical and psychosocial interventions, but sufficient residual symptoms persist to justify a continued Risk Rating of 3; ***or:*** (2) The patient's withdrawal symptoms, although initially compatible with a Risk Rating of 2, have intensified despite appropriate treatment; ***or:*** (3) The patient's withdrawal symptoms, while initially compatible with a Risk Rating of 4, have improved sufficiently in response to treatment to warrant a reduction to a Risk Rating of 3.	rehabilitation program or other suitable psychosocial interventions (*see Appendix B*). Transportation to return the patient to his or her home and overnight supervision should be arranged. Alternatively, residential support may be indicated if there is a significant likelihood that the patient will not complete detoxification or enter into continuing addiction treatment.	**Concurrent OMT** The OMT patient who has a Risk Rating of **3** requires continuation of opioid maintenance medications, such as methadone or buprenorphine, during and after withdrawal from alcohol, along with assessment for dose adjustment, counseling services to assess and address readiness to change and relapse issues, and random urine testing. During detoxification from alcohol, opioid maintenance medications should be provided either by the detoxification program or through coordination with the patient's Level I outpatient OMT program.
Risk Rating = 4 (Severe risk) A Risk Rating of **4** in Dimension 1 indicates that the patient is incapacitated, with severe signs and symptoms of withdrawal. Such a patient is in imminent danger from either the continued use of alcohol (through liver failure, gastrointestinal bleed, fetal death, etc.) or the abrupt discontinuation of use (through withdrawal seizures, delirium, or acute hallucinosis). **Initial Assessment** The patient with a Risk Rating of **4** evidences one of the following: (1) The patient has clouding of the sensorium or confusion, or new onset of hallucinations, or has experienced a seizure, or is not able to fully comprehend instructions; which generally is associated with a CIWA-Ar score greater than 20*;	**Service Needs** A Risk Rating of **4** in Dimension 1 indicates a need for high-intensity intoxication monitoring or detoxification services, with medical monitoring and management more often than hourly. **Treatment Interventions** Benzodiazepine medication should be administered. Short- or long-acting agents may be appropriate, depending on the circumstances (e.g., short-acting and nonhepatically metabolized agents such as oxazepam or lorazepam are preferable in the presence of hepatic insufficiency)	**Appropriate Level of Care or Setting** The patient with a Risk Rating of **4** should be placed in a Level IV-D medically managed intensive inpatient detoxification program, which is an organized hospital addiction service. In the absence of such a service, an organized medical or psychiatric service in a hospital under the direction of an addiction medicine specialist may be used. If the patient requires medically monitored and nurse-managed

or: (2) The patient has severe anxiety and a moderate to severe tremor. He or she also may be withdrawing from a substance other than alcohol. The patient would otherwise have had a Risk Rating of **3**, except that he or she evidences one or more of the following problems, which pose a major impediment to detoxification at a less intensive level of care: a. The patient has severe destabilizing medical problems, such as hepatitis, or persistent vomiting, as from gastritis or pancreatitis. b. Symptoms of a co-occurring psychiatric disorder (such as a mood, anxiety, or attention deficit disorder) are severe. c. The patient's past attempts to stop drinking were marked by seizures or delirium tremens. d. The patient is not cooperative or reliable, to an extent that places him or her at imminent risk of harm. e. The patient requires medical monitoring for more than 5 hours a day. **Concurrent OMT** For patients undergoing concurrent OMT, a Risk Rating of **4** is compatible with varying degrees of stability or instability of the dose, varying degrees of symptoms of opioid withdrawal, and/ or concurrent illicit use of opioids. **Reassessment** On reassessment after initiation of treatment, the patient with a Risk Rating of **4** evidences one of the following: (1) The patient's symptoms are currently improving as a result of the medical and psychosocial interventions, but sufficient residual symptoms persist to justify a continued Risk Rating of **4**; ***or:*** (2) The patient's withdrawal symptoms, although initially compatible with a Risk Rating of **3**, have intensified despite appropriate treatment.	Parenteral hydration as well as other appropriate supportive medications should be available. The patient should be closely monitored (at least several times a day, or hourly in the presence of delirium or substantial elevation of vital signs) through the use of the CIWA-Ar* or equivalent instrument. The dose should be repeated, using a symptom-triggered or time-driven protocol, with a symptom-driven override/rescue protocol in place. As soon as he or she is medically stable, the patient should be offered immediate access to, and simultaneous participation in, a rehabilitation program or other suitable psychosocial interventions (*see Appendix B*).	mental health services (with a Risk Rating of **3** or higher in Dimension 3), moderately high-intensity detoxification can be provided in a mental health setting with ongoing case management to coordinate care. **Concurrent OMT** The OMT patient who has a Risk Rating of **4** generally requires continuation of opioid maintenance medications, such as methadone or buprenorphine, during detoxification. However, on an individualized basis when withdrawal symptoms include delirium, consideration should be given to a temporary opioid agonist taper during the period of altered mental status, with resumption of opioid maintenance when those symptoms resolve. During hospitalization, opioid maintenance medications should be provided. Following detoxification, the OMT patient who has a Risk Rating of **4** requires continuation of opioid maintenance medications, such as methadone or buprenorphine, along with assessment for dose adjustment, counseling services to assess and address readiness to change and relapse issues, and random urine testing. Such a patient should continue in a Level I OMT program once he or she is stable enough to do so.

****Note:*** While CIWA-Ar scores are widely used and may be somewhat helpful as an imprecise general guide to the overall severity of withdrawal symptoms, they should not be regarded as comprehensive (e.g., they do not reflect vital signs and do not take into account the relative weight of particular features of withdrawal, such as tremulousness, confusion, psychosis, etc.). The presence of particular clinical signs and symptoms (as outlined in this text) should be taken as red flags and used as a *more important guide* to treatment service and level of care decisions. CIWA-Ar scores are more useful as a *monitoring tool* to track the changing severity of withdrawal (up or down) for a particular patient over time (e.g., in response to treatment).

CHAPTER 5

Strategies for Preventing and Managing Relapse

ASSESSING THE RISK OF RELAPSE OR CONTINUED USE

The primary goal of treatment for alcohol use disorders is the interruption of alcohol use and the prevention of continued use. Among the major challenges confronting alcohol-dependent patients who have stopped drinking is the prevention of relapse to alcohol use, which is a risk even with a successful treatment intervention.

The term *lapse* (sometimes referred to as a *slip*) refers to an initial episode of alcohol or other drug use after a period of abstinence. A lapse usually is impulsive and involves a brief period of use. Most lapses are of short duration, with relatively minor consequences, and are marked by the patient's desire to return to abstinence. However, a lapse also can progress to a full-blown relapse (marked by loss of control) of varying proportions. The effects of the initial lapse are mediated by the individual's affective and cognitive state, as well as the response of caregivers and others.

Although some individuals in *relapse* return to pretreatment levels of active addiction, others use alcohol (or other drugs) problematically but do not return to previous levels of abuse, and thus suffer fewer harmful effects as a result. Patients in relapse vary in the quantity and frequency of their substance use, as well as the accompanying medical and psychosocial sequelae.

Continued use implies just that—continued use of nonprescribed psychoactive substances including alcohol without having first achieved a period of stability or sobriety, regardless of whether an intervention has taken place. Abstinence in a protected environment (e.g., a residential treatment or incarceration), followed by a return to drinking, is more appropriately considered "continued use" rather than "relapse," as is continued use while in outpatient treatment (e.g., drinking between outpatient therapy sessions).

Continued problem potential addresses the issues of co-occurring mental health problems that are related to substance use. For example, a psychotic, paranoid individual who is fearful of being poisoned and thus fails to take his or her medication would be described as having a "high relapse or continued use potential" and may also be at high risk for becoming acutely psychotic and/or increasingly paranoid. By the nature of the mental health disorder, such a person is at high risk of relapse to substance use.

Neurophysiology of Relapse

Alcohol influences several neurochemical systems in the brain, including the γ-aminobutyric acid (GABA), glutamate, dopamine, and opiate systems (Koob et al., 1998). The GABA and glutamate systems are primarily involved with alcohol stimulation, sedation, and intoxication, as well as many symptoms of alcohol withdrawal. The dopamine and opiate systems are involved with reinforcement, reward, some aspects of craving, sustained use of alcohol, and potential relapse after prolonged abstinence in the dependent person (Anton, 2008b).

Acute alcohol use stimulates neurons in the ventral tegmental area of the brain, inducing the release of dopamine in the nucleus accumbens, an area of the brain that mediates reward, pleasure, and the assignment of salience to important environmental stimuli (Fig. 5-1). This effect may be enhanced by environmental cues that are associated with alcohol ingestion. Using brain-imaging techniques, investigators have shown that the nucleus accumbens of persons with alcohol dependence—but not social drinkers—is activated by such alcohol cues (Heinz et al., 2004; Myrick et al., 2004).

Several other neuronal pathways that are influenced by alcohol modulate this dopaminergic pathway. Low doses of alcohol stimulate the glutamate system, which enhances dopaminergic activity and leads to arousal and increased energy. In contrast, higher doses of alcohol inhibit glutamate and augment GABA neurotransmission, suppressing dopaminergic activity and leading to sedation, among other effects. These pathways are further modulated by endogenous opioid-like protein neurotransmitters, enkephalins and β-endorphin. Such "endogenous opioids" are thought to be released during alcohol intoxication and may contribute to alcohol addiction by inhibiting GABA pathways and enhancing dopaminergic signaling (Anton, 2008b). Plasma β-endorphin levels rise significantly in response to alcohol in high risk but not in low risk drinkers (Gianoulakis, 1990). Interestingly, mice without mu-opiate receptors do not self-administer alcohol (Roberts et al., 2000).

Precipitants of Relapse

Relapse rarely is caused by any single factor and often is the result of an interaction of individual, situational, physiologic, and sociocultural factors (Dimeff & Marlatt, 1995; Marlatt, Barrett, & Daley, 1999). It is best viewed as a dynamic process in which the patient's readiness to change interacts with other external and internal factors (Marlatt, 1996a,b).

Specific precipitants of relapse vary substantially from one experience to the next, even in the same individual. Catalano and colleagues (1988) reviewed the literature on relapse in alcoholism, heroin addiction, and smoking and classified relapse precipitants in three categories: (1) pretreatment factors, such as the degree of substance dependence or psychiatric impairment; (2) treatment factors, such as the type and duration of treatment; and (3) posttreatment factors, such as family supports or social skills. Brain chemistry also contributes, and various brain chemicals have been implicated in mediating alcohol's pleasant effects and in contributing to the development of tolerance to and craving for alcohol.

Attributing causality is even more complex in patients with comorbid substance use and psychiatric disorders. In a survey of more than 100 such patients, Daley, Salloum et al. (1998) asked them to identify the factors contributing to their relapse. The five factors identified most often as contributing to relapse were inability to manage stress or negative emotional states

(69%), interpersonal conflicts with family or others (29%), poor adherence to professional treatment (25%), negative thinking (11%), and low motivation to change (10%).

Clinical Picture

Although relapse can be the result of an impulsive act, it also is possible that attitudinal, emotional, cognitive, and/or behavioral changes are evident days or weeks before the actual ingestion of substances. Patients are better prepared for the challenges of recovery if they understand that relapse occurs in a larger context and that warning signs often precede an actual lapse or relapse. Such warning signs may be overt and obvious, such as stopping or reducing treatment sessions or self-help meetings without discussing the decision with a therapist or sponsor, or they may be less overt, as when a patient experiences a significant increase in cravings for alcohol or other drugs. Or they may be less subjectively apparent, as when a patient undergoes increased stress without noticing attendant loss of stability or increased vulnerability. Patients in treatment for the first time can benefit from a discussion of common relapse warning signs, as identified by others in recovery (Daley, 2000; Marlatt, 1985).

One of the values of the involvement of helping others (e.g., a professional counselor, a 12-step sponsor, or a trusted friend or family member) is assistance in the early identification of warning signs before the actual occurrence of relapse.

Relapse is more likely to occur as the result of inadequate coping skills than the high-risk situation itself, so the patient's coping skills should be assessed and any deficits targeted for clinical intervention (Marlatt, 1985; Connors, Longabaugh et al., 1996).

For some patients, identifying risk factors and developing new coping strategies for each is inadequate because they can identify many risk factors. Such patients need help in taking a more global approach to recovery and may need to learn broader problem-solving skills.

NONPHARMACOLOGIC APPROACHES TO RELAPSE PREVENTION

General Strategies

The following general strategies are drawn from various models of relapse prevention and other treatment models that incorporate relapse issues.

Strategy 1: Identify Environmental Cues That Act as Relapse Triggers

Identifying the environmental cues associated with use is critical, and can lead to the development of a relapse prevention plan through the use of such techniques as cue avoidance, cue desensitization, and stimulus control. Environmental triggers, sometimes characterized as "people, places, and things," are usually so interwoven into the lives of patients with substance use disorders that they do not easily or intuitively identify them. Moreover, patients often have difficulty in appreciating the causality associated with environmental cues and opportunities for access to substances. Many have the impression that relapse occurs spontaneously, without a specific cause or explanation. Analyzing antecedent events with a "time lapse photography" approach is a particularly useful intervention.

Strategy 2: Identify Environmental Stressors That Act as Relapse Triggers

Identifying such stressors as early as possible, as a part of the comprehensive assessment, can help both the patient and clinician determine those stress triggers likely to precipitate relapse or continued use. Identifying such triggers can lead to the identification of those coping skills most needed by the patient and initiation of interventions to develop them. An efficient way to identify high relapse risk stressors as triggers is for the clinician to complete a "relapse trigger inventory" (see Chapter 6), which is a substance use disorder expansion of the *Diagnostic and Statistical Manual of Mental Disorders, Fourth Edition, Text Revision (DSM-IV-TR),* Axis IV, Psychosocial and Environmental Stressors.

Strategy 3: Help the Patient Identify Feelings and Manage Negative Emotional States

Interventions that help patients develop appropriate skills to cope with or manage negative emotional states can reduce the risk of relapse but must be tailored to the situation of each patient. For example, strategies for dealing with the depression that accompanies the realization that addiction has caused havoc in one's life may differ from interventions designed to address the clinical symptoms that accompany bipolar or major depressive illness.

Similarly, interventions to help the patient who occasionally becomes angry and seeks solace in alcohol will differ from interventions for the patient who is chronically angry. The former may need help in expressing anger appropriately rather than suppressing it, whereas the chronically angry patient is more likely to benefit from cognitive techniques that help challenge and change angry thoughts. Interventions for patients who report feelings of chronic boredom, emptiness, or joylessness similarly depend on the specific nature of the emotional state (Marlatt & Gordon, 1985).

Strategy 4: Help the Patient Work Toward a More Balanced Lifestyle

Development of a healthy lifestyle is important in reducing the stress that renders patients vulnerable to relapse. Lifestyle can be assessed by evaluating patterns of daily activities; sources of stress and stressful life events; daily hassles and uplifts; the balance between wants (activities engaged in for pleasure or self-fulfillment) and "shoulds" (external demands); health, exercise and relaxation patterns; interpersonal activities; and religious beliefs (Marlatt & Gordon, 1985). Helping patients develop positive habits or substitute healthy indulgences (such as jogging, meditation, relaxation, exercise, hobbies, or creative tasks) for an addictive disorder can help to balance their lifestyles.

Strategy 5: Help the Patient Understand Craving

Volkow and Fowler (2000) hypothesize that the dopamine stimulation that occurs with long-term alcohol or drug use leads to disruption of brain circuitry involved in regulating drives. This disruption, in turn, leads to a conditioned response to the stimulus (craving), which leads to compulsive use of the substance.

To help patients understand and manage this process, clinicians can provide information about cues that trigger craving, as well as coping strategies. For example, monitoring and recording cravings, associated thoughts, and outcomes in a daily log or journal can help patients become more aware of cues and cravings.

Strategy 6: Help the Patient Manage Craving

Useful cognitive interventions include helping the patient change his or her thoughts about craving, challenging euphoric recall, talking oneself through the craving, identifying the negative consequences of use (immediate and delayed) and the positive benefits of abstaining, and delaying the decision to use.

Behavioral interventions include avoiding, leaving, or changing situations that trigger or worsen craving; redirecting activities or becoming involved in pleasant activities; obtaining help or support from others by admitting and talking about cravings and hearing how others have survived them; attending self-help support group meetings; or using anticraving medications (Drummond, Litten et al., 2000; Li, 2000).

Patients' understanding that craving need not inevitably lead to a return to use, and that cravings not reinforced by use tend to become less intense and less frequent over time, can render these interventions more effective.

Strategy 7: Prepare the Patient to Interrupt Lapses and Relapses as Quickly as Possible

Patients should have an emergency plan to address a lapse so that a full-blown relapse can be avoided. However, if relapse does occur, the patient needs strategies to interrupt it. Intervention strategies should be based on the severity of the patient's lapse or relapse, the presence of coping mechanisms, and his or her history of relapse. Helpful interventions include asking family, Alcoholic's Anonymous (AA) sponsors, friends, or professionals for help; carrying an emergency card with names and phone numbers of others who can be called for support; or carrying a reminder card that gives specific instructions as to what to do if a lapse or relapse occurs (Daley, 2000). Marlatt (1985) recommends developing a relapse "contract" with the patient that outlines specific steps to be taken in the event of a relapse (the goal of such a contract is to formalize or reinforce the patient's commitment to change).

Once a relapsed patient is stabilized, analyzing the cues that triggered the relapse, as well as the strategies that were effective in interrupting it, is a valuable process that can aid in ongoing recovery. Through this process, the patient may be able to identify warning signs that preceded actual substance use, as well as the relevant risk factors. Such a process also can help the patient reframe the relapse as a learning experience.

Strategy 8: Help the Patient Improve His or Her Interpersonal Relationships and Develop a Recovery Support System

Positive family and social supports generally enhance recovery. Families are more likely to provide such support if they are engaged in the treatment process and have an opportunity to ask questions, share their concerns and experiences, and learn practical coping strategies as well as behaviors to avoid (Daley & Raskin, 1991).

Some patients find it helpful to put their action plan into writing. Such an action plan might address the following issues: how to communicate about and deal with relapse warning signs and high-risk situations, how to interrupt a lapse, how to intervene if a relapse occurs, and the importance of exploring all the details of a lapse/relapse after the patient is stable so that it can be used as a learning experience. A plan can make both the recovering person and the family feel more in control, even when faced with the possibility of an actual relapse.

PHARMACOLOGIC APPROACHES TO RELAPSE PREVENTION

Pharmacotherapies are becoming a standard component of the relapse prevention and management armamentarium. While not indicated for every patient, they are an important component of care for many individuals.

The development of these medicines has been facilitated by advances in the neurosciences that have implicated several target neurotransmitter systems, such as those within the corticomesolimbic dopamine (CMDA) pathway, which mediate alcohol's reinforcing effects associated with its abuse liability. Additionally, it is now known that some individuals may possess a biological predisposition to the disease. These biologically vulnerable persons can be expected to benefit from specific adjunctive medication targeted toward correcting or ameliorating the underlying abnormalities.

The treatment of alcohol dependence also has been advanced by development of new models as well as broader therapeutic objectives. For example, an important model is that, with appropriate pharmacotherapy, it is possible to initiate treatment for alcohol dependence while the patient is still drinking heavily and at the point of maximum crisis and help-seeking behavior (Johnson et al., 2003). To broaden access to treatment, effective but brief and standardized behavioral treatments have been developed that can be provided more readily in the general practice setting (Johnson, 2008; Pettinati, Gastfriend, Dong, Kranzler, & O'Malley, 2009). Finally, it is now more widely accepted that although abstinence remains the ultimate goal in treating alcohol-dependent individuals, reducing the frequency of heavy drinking has the potential to reduce the potential for alcohol-related consequences and improve the patient's quality of life (Johnson, 2008; Pettinati et al., 2009).

FDA–Approved Medications

Naltrexone and acamprosate have shown mixed results in clinical trials. Oral naltrexone and extended-release injectable naltrexone have demonstrated efficacy at treating alcohol dependence, but their treatment effect size is small and more research is needed to compare the effects of different doses on drinking outcome. Acamprosate has demonstrated efficacy for treating alcohol dependence in European trials. In U.S. trials, acamprosate has not proved efficacious. Researchers continue to explore which groups of alcohol-dependent individuals would benefit most from treatment with naltrexone or acamprosate. Combinations of acamprosate and naltrexone have shown efficacy for treating alcohol dependence in one European study, but not in a multisite U.S. study (Johnson, 2007, 2008; National Institute on Alcohol Abuse and Alcoholism [NIAAA], 2008).

Disulfiram is an aversive agent that does not diminish craving for alcohol. Disulfiram is most effective when given to those who are highly compliant or who are receiving their medication under supervision (Johnson, 2008; NIAAA, 2008).

Off-label and Experimental Uses

Of the agents that have not been FDA-approved for the treatment of alcoholism, topiramate is among the most promising, with a medium effect size in clinical trials. Another promising medication, baclofen, has shown efficacy in small trials. Serotonergic agents such as selective serotonin reuptake inhibitors (SSRIs) and the serotonin-3 receptor antagonist, ondansetron, appear to be efficacious only in patients with certain genetic subtypes of alcoholism (Anton, 2008a; Garbutt, West, Carey, Lohr, & Crews, 1999; Johnson, 2008; NIAAA, 2008).

As the number of available pharmacotherapies grows, practitioners need to carefully consider the indications and contraindications for each. Considerations include patient factors, medication factors, integration with psychosocial treatments, methods for assessing and enhancing motivation and adherence, and potential interactions with other drugs.

Pharmacotherapies can be employed at any level of care, including a medical office setting, that does not meet the criteria for Level I outpatient services (i.e., an organized addiction service). Initiation of antiaddiction medication in the context of the high-intensity services typically offered by medically monitored treatment can be of considerable help in reinforcing medication adherence. Residential/inpatient monitoring may be necessary to establish the lead-in period of abstinence recommended as a prelude to initiation of antiaddiction medications (as in a step-down from withdrawal or a step-up from a less intensive level of care). Initiation of medication, including monitoring for and management of transient side effects, may be an added indication for a medically monitored inpatient (III.7) level of care.

Wherever they are given, pharmacotherapies should be used in combination with appropriate psychosocial treatments in order to enhance patient outcomes. Patients who previously failed to respond to psychosocial approaches alone are particularly strong candidates for medication treatment. A relatively rare exception involves those few cases where use of nonpharmacologic therapies would place the patient at risk for premature termination of treatment. In such cases, the pharmacotherapy should be continued, but offered in combination with motivational enhancement strategies to help the patient accept the value of other psychosocial treatments. Conversely, there might be other situations, also rare, in which the use of pharmacotherapy combined with psychosocial treatment is indicated but the patient is resistant to using medication and any insistence on its use would place the patient at risk for premature termination of treatment. Again, psychosocial treatments should be continued, but offered in combination with motivational enhancement strategies to help the patient accept the value of pharmacotherapy (NIAAA, 2008; Swift, 2007).

Regardless of the medication used, patients who have a goal of abstinence, or who can abstain even for a few days prior to starting the medication, are likely to have better outcomes. (This underscores the importance of establishing individual goals with each patient.) Some patients may not be willing to endorse abstinence as a goal, especially at first. If a patient with alcohol dependence agrees to reduce drinking substantially, it's best to engage him or her in that goal while continuing to note that abstinence remains the optimal outcome (Anton et al., 2006; Johnson, 2008; NIAAA, 2008).

Acamprosate

Acamprosate (Campral®) acts on the GABA and glutamate neurotransmitter systems and is thought to reduce symptoms of protracted abstinence such as insomnia, anxiety, restlessness, and dysphoria (Johnson, 2008).

Formulation and Dose Acamprosate is available in enteric-coated delayed-release tablets and generally is given three times a day.

Mechanism of Action Although the precise mechanism(s) of action of acamprosate remains to be fully elucidated, it appears that it involves beneficial modulation of the glutamatergic neurotransmitter system, including antagonism of the mGLu5 metabotropic glutamate receptor, to counteract the imbalance between the glutamatergic and GABAergic systems associated with chronic alcohol exposure and alcohol withdrawal (Johnson, 2008; Scott, Figgitt, Keam, & Waugh, 2005; Swift, 2007).

Acamprosate is thought to share some of the cellular actions of taurine, affecting GABA and glutaminergic receptors in the nucleus accumbens, a brain region that may be responsible for the reinforcing effects of alcohol consumption. It also may suppress excitation-induced calcium entry that results from chronic alcohol exposure, thereby altering the conformation of the *N*-methyl-D-aspartate receptors. The glutamatergic hypothesis of acamprosate's mechanism of action may provide a unifying hypothesis that can explain the diverse neurochemical effects of acamprosate (Boothby & Doering, 2005; De Witte, Littleton, Parot, & Koob, 2005; Johnson, 2008).

Safety Acamprosate is well tolerated and has limited side effects (principally transient diarrhea, which occurs in approximately 10%; Williams, 2005). No interactions have been reported related to concomitant use of acamprosate with alcohol, diazepam (Valium®), disulfiram (Antabuse®), or imipramine (Tofranil®). Patients with alcohol dependence can safely continue to use acamprosate during a relapse (NIAAA, 2008; Williams, 2005).

Efficacy Acamprosate increases the proportion of dependent drinkers who maintain abstinence for several weeks to months, a result demonstrated in multiple European studies and confirmed by a metaanalysis of 17 clinical trials (Mann, 2004). The metaanalysis reported that 36% of patients taking acamprosate were continuously abstinent at 6 months, compared with 23% of those taking a placebo. However, two large U.S. trials failed to confirm the efficacy of acamprosate (Anton et al., 2006; Mason, 2006).

A reason for the discrepancy between European and U.S. findings may be that patients in European trials had more severe dependence than patients in U.S. trials (Anton et al., 2006; Mann, 2004), a factor consistent with preclinical studies showing that acamprosate has a greater effect in animals with a prolonged history of dependence (Rimondini, Arlinde et al., 2002). In addition, before starting medication, most patients in European trials had been abstinent longer than patients in U.S. trials (Mason & Ownby, 2000; NIAAA, 2008).

Patient Selection Acamprosate may be particularly useful in patients who are strongly committed to abstinence (Johnson, 2008; Mason, 2006), as well as in those with hepatic impairment and/or liver disease (Scott et al., 2005).

Cautions and Contraindications Patients with moderate renal insufficiency should receive a reduced dose (333 mg three times a day [TID]), while those with advanced renal insufficiency should not be given acamprosate (Graham, Wodak, & Whelan, 2002).

Use in Pregnancy Acamprosate is classified in FDA pregnancy category C (adverse effects on the fetus in animal studies, but no human trials have been conducted).

Use in Patients with Co-Occurring Medical or Psychiatric Disorders
Acamprosate may be taken safely by patients with liver dysfunction but not advanced kidney disease (Graham et al., 2002). There is no incompatibility with other medications for psychiatric conditions.

Clinical Recommendation

Based on the weight of evidence for its effectiveness, acamprosate is recommended as an FDA-approved pharmacotherapy for the treatment of alcohol dependence in appropriately selected patients and in conjunction with psychosocial therapies (NIAAA, 2008).

Disulfiram

Disulfiram (Antabuse®) interferes with degradation of alcohol, resulting in accumulation of acetaldehyde, which in turn produces a very unpleasant reaction including flushing, nausea, and palpitations if the patient drinks alcohol. While disulfiram does not specifically block craving, if taken regularly, it may simplify the daily struggle against urges toward alcohol (O'Brien, 2006).

Formulation and Dose Disulfiram is available in 250- and 500-mg oral tablets (Antabuse®). The clinical use of the sulfoxide metabolite of disulfiram that directly antagonizes the activity of aldehyde dehydrogenase (ALDH) can eliminate much of the variability in response observed with the drug.

Because the risk of side effects and of toxic hazards increases with the dose, the daily dose prescribed in the U.S. has been limited to 250 to 500 mg/day. (The requirement that disulfiram undergo bioactivation before it can inhibit ALDH [Yourick & Faiman, 1991] may explain the need for a higher dose in some patients. At the dose that is used clinically, faulty bioactivation in some individuals can yield too low a concentration of the active metabolite to inhibit ALDH.)

Mechanism of Action Disulfiram blocks the enzyme acetaldehyde dehydrogenase so that, if the patient takes a drink, the metabolite acetaldehyde accumulates, causing a very unpleasant flushing reaction known as the disulfiram-ethanol reaction (DER).

The DER generally varies in intensity both with the dose of disulfiram and with the volume of alcohol ingested. In its mild form, the syndrome includes warmness and flushing of the skin, especially that of the upper chest and face; increased heart rate; palpitations; and decreased blood pressure. Nausea, vomiting, shortness of breath, sweating, dizziness, blurred vision, and confusion also can occur.

Most reactions last about 30 minutes and are self-limited. However, more severe reactions do occur, involving marked tachycardia, hypotension, bradycardia, or even cardiac arrest secondary to vagal stimulation associated with retching or vomiting. Cardiovascular collapse, congestive failure, and convulsions have been reported. Although severe reactions usually are associated with high doses of disulfiram (more than 500 mg/day), combined with more than 2 ounces of alcohol, deaths have occurred at lower doses and after a single drink (Lindros, Stowell et al., 1981; Peachey, Brien et al., 1981; Peachey, Maglana et al., 1981; Sellers, Naranjo, & Peachey, 1981).

This effect is the basis for the admonition to avoid alcohol consumption for at least 2 weeks after the final dose of disulfiram.

Despite the possibility of underdosing, some clinicians prescribe a 125-mg dose in order to minimize the risk of a severe DER or even a mild DER in response to accidental exposure to a low dose of alcohol.

Safety Common side effects of disulfiram include drowsiness, lethargy, and fatigue. Other more serious adverse effects, such as optic neuritis, peripheral neuropathy, and hepatotoxicity, are rare (Chick, 1999). Although uncommon, potentially severe features of the disulfiram ethanol reaction can include myocardial infarction, congestive heart failure, respiratory depression, and even death (Chick, 1999; Doering, 1999; NIAAA, 2008).

In addition to the toxicity caused by accumulation of acetaldehyde, adverse effects of disulfiram or its metabolites can occur as a result of multiple drug interactions. For example, disulfiram reduces clearance rates of chlordiazepoxide (Librium®) and diazepam (Valium®), although benzodiazepines that do not require hydroxylation before excretion (such as lorazepam [Ativan®] and oxazepam [Serax®]) are not altered. Disulfiram also can reduce the clearance, increase the elimination half-life, and lead to higher peak plasma levels of desipramine (Norpramin®) and imipramine (Tofranil®) (Ciraulo, Barnhill, & Boxenbaum, 1985). Clearance of phenytoin (Dilantin®) and warfarin (Coumadin®) is reduced, and dose adjustments are required to avoid adverse effects (Hoyumpa & Schenker, 1982; Sellers et al., 1981).

Efficacy Although the efficacy of disulfiram in the prevention or limitation of relapse in alcoholics has been supported in some studies, it has not been clearly shown in methodologically rigorous research (Johnson, 2008; NIAAA, 2008; Swift, 2007). For example, most studies undertaken before the last decade failed to include measures of compliance or adequate controls, both of which now are considered essential elements in evaluating the efficacy of such a medication (Johnson, 2008; Kranzler, Mason, Pettinati, & Anton, 1997).

An evidence report from the Agency for Healthcare Research and Quality (Garbutt et al., 1999) concluded that the four placebo-controlled randomized clinical trials of oral disulfiram produced mixed results. Although disulfiram was shown to reduce frequency of drinking days in two trials, in neither study did it improve relapse rates compared with placebo. Two studies that examined patient compliance with oral disulfiram showed it to be low (Fuller & Gordis, 2004; Williams, 2005), and a third study had a 46% dropout rate (Laaksonen, Koski-Jännes, Salaspuro, Ahtinen, & Alho, 2008). These methodologic limitations and mixed results make it difficult to state clearly how many patients benefit from disulfiram.

Patient Selection There are no evidence-based guidelines to identify patients for whom disulfiram is most likely to have a beneficial effect (NIAAA, 2008). However, there is some consensus that it may be useful in situations in which moderate impulsivity is likely to be deterred by the imposition of more concrete, immediate, and predictable consequences to drinking; in a patient who has the goal of abstinence; or in situations in which consequences of drinking are considered imminently dangerous and/or potentially devastating (Johnson, 2008).

Disulfiram should be avoided if abstinence is unlikely because of the patient's severe impulsivity, unpredictability, or subjective intention to continue drinking. Controversy surrounds the ethics of prescribing disulfiram to anyone except a patient who wishes to use it to achieve abstinence, and who has no psychological or medical contraindications (Johnson, 2008). Nevertheless, disulfiram has been incorporated as a mandatory element in some court-ordered treatment programs.

Cautions and Contraindications Disulfiram is contraindicated in patients who have psychosis or cardiovascular disease, as well as those who have recently received metronidazole (which causes an additive acetaldehyde accumulation in the presence of alcohol) or ingested alcohol.

Because of the potential for a severe alcohol–disulfiram interactions, disulfiram is *not* recommended for patients with severe pulmonary disease, chronic renal failure, or diabetes or those older than 60 years. It also is not recommended in patients with peripheral neuropathy, seizures, or cirrhosis with portal hypertension.

Patients should be warned carefully about the hazards of disulfiram, including the need to avoid over-the-counter preparations containing alcohol or drugs that interact adversely with disulfiram. A warning also should be provided about the potential for a DER precipitated by alcohol used in food preparation (NIAAA, 2008).

Use in Pregnancy Disulfiram is classified in FDA pregnancy category C (adverse effects on the fetus in animal studies, but no human trials have been conducted).

Use in Patients with Co-Occurring Medical or Psychiatric Disorders The inhibition of dopamine beta hydroxylase (DBH) by disulfiram and its metabolite produce increased dopamine levels. The exacerbation of psychotic symptoms in schizophrenics and occasionally their appearance in others, as well as the development of depression, may be linked to this action.

As with the neuropathic effects, the psychiatric effects are uncommon and may depend for their appearance on higher doses of disulfiram. Patients with low cerebrospinal fluid, DBH activity is more likely to develop dysphoric or psychotic symptoms in response to disulfiram (Major et al., 1979; Sellers et al., 1981).

Clinical Recommendation Based on the weight of evidence for its effectiveness, disulfiram should probably be considered, in combination with suitable adherence enhancement procedures, in patients who are motivated toward abstinence and not so impulsive that they are likely to drink while taking the medication.

Naltrexone (Oral Formulation)

Naltrexone is an opiate receptor antagonist with no intrinsic agonist properties. Naltrexone blocks opioid receptors that are involved in the rewarding effects of drinking alcohol and the craving for alcohol (Anton et al., 2006).

One factor that appears important to naltrexone's effectiveness is adherence (Anton, 2008b). In general, patients being treated for alcohol dependence demonstrate low rates of medication adherence. Nonadherence poses the additional problem that, if a patient on oral naltrexone wants to resume drinking or using drugs, he or she can readily discontinue the medication and experience the full effect of alcohol or other drugs.

Formulation and Dose Naltrexone is available in 50-mg oral tablets (ReVia®, Depade®); also see the discussion of the extended-release injectable formulation.

The recommended dose of oral naltrexone is 50 mg per day, given in a single dose (Williams, 2005). Although there are no published clinical trials in which the dose of naltrexone was varied systematically, a laboratory-based study in which alcohol was administered (McCaul, Wand, Wand, Rohde, & Lee, 2000) showed that pretreatment with 100 mg of the drug had significantly greater effects than did a 50-mg dose. As might be expected, the higher naltrexone dose produced higher levels of its major metabolite, 6-α-naltrexol. Higher metabolite levels of naltrexone were associated with significantly reduced positive effects of alcohol after high-dose alcohol administration. This and other suggestive evidence has led to an emerging consensus that 100 mg may be the preferred dose (it was, for example, the dose chosen for the COMBINE study [Anton et al., 2006]).

Mechanism of Action Naltrexone is believed to work by blocking mu-opioid receptors, thereby reducing the reinforcing effects of alcohol and leading to decreased feelings of intoxication and fewer cravings (Williams, 2005). O'Malley, Jaffe, Rode, and Rounsaville (1996) found that naltrexone reduced craving for alcohol, alcohol's reinforcing properties, the experience of intoxication, and the chances of continued drinking after a slip. Study subjects who drank while taking naltrexone reported less euphoria, which may indicate that naltrexone blocked the contribution of the endogenous opioid system to alcohol's "priming effect" (Volpicelli, Watson, King, Sherman, & O'Brien, 1995).

Safety Naltrexone generally is well tolerated, although it does have the potential to precipitate severe opioid withdrawal in opioid-dependent patients (Williams, 2005).

Medication side effects have been a problem in less than 10% of patients, with nausea and (occasionally) vomiting the most commonly reported. The rate seems to be higher in individuals who begin naltrexone while still actively drinking alcohol (Johnson, 2008).

Studies using seven times the normal dose of naltrexone in obese subjects produced elevated liver enzymes, leading to an FDA Black Box warning. However, this is potentially misleading because naltrexone actually protects the liver from alcohol, which is demonstrably more hepatotoxic. Most studies have found that patients have elevated liver enzymes on entry into the study, but the group randomized to naltrexone has liver function moving toward normal after several weeks or months on naltrexone because of the reduction in drinking (O'Brien, 2006).

Efficacy Oral naltrexone reduces relapse to heavy drinking, defined as four or more drinks per day for women and five or more for men (Bouza, Angeles, Muñoz, & Amate, 2004; NIAAA, 2008; Srisurapanont & Jarusuraisin, 2005a,b). It reduces the relapse risk during the first 3 months by about 36% (about 28% of patients taking naltrexone relapse versus about 43% of those taking a placebo relapse [Srisurapanont & Jarusuraisin, 2005a]). Thus, it is especially helpful for curbing consumption in patients who have drinking "slips." It is less effective in maintaining abstinence (Bouza et al., 2004; Srisurapanont & Jarusuraisin, 2005a,b).

Clinical trials beginning in the 1980s at the Philadelphia VA Medical Center demonstrated that the effect of naltrexone seems to reside in its ability to block the reward from alcohol. It also reduces craving for alcohol. Most studies have shown that there is a significant decrease in drinking and increased abstinence among people randomized to naltrexone as compared to a group randomized to placebo (O'Brien, 2006).

In a systematic review (Srisurapanont & Jarusuraisin, 2005b) of 11 double-blind, placebo-controlled trials, researchers found that oral naltrexone reduced short-term relapse rates in patients with alcohol dependence when combined with psychosocial treatments. Short-term outcomes in favor of naltrexone included fewer patients relapsing to alcohol dependence (38%

vs. 60% with placebo), fewer patients returning to drinking (61% vs. 69%), reduced cravings for alcohol, and fewer drinking days (Srisurapanont & Jarusuraisin, 2005a). The data showed one relapse was prevented for every five patients treated with naltrexone (i.e., number needed to treat [NNT] = 5).

Randomized controlled trials that looked at longer-term outcomes reported mixed results. In a systematic review (Garbutt et al., 1999) of three studies assessing medium-term outcomes (6 to 12 months), researchers found no difference between oral naltrexone and placebo groups. In addition, a large trial (Krystal et al., 2001) comparing outcomes of three therapy groups—12 months of naltrexone therapy, 3 months of naltrexone followed by 9 months of placebo, and 12 months of placebo—found no significant differences among the groups in the number of days to relapse, number of drinking days, or number of drinks per drinking day. Although there is good evidence supporting short-term benefit with naltrexone, the evidence for longer-term use is less compelling (Williams, 2005).

O'Malley, Jaffe, and colleagues (1996) found that the beneficial effects of naltrexone diminished gradually over time. Similarly, Anton and colleagues (1999, 2000) found that oral naltrexone was superior to placebo in the percentage of days abstinent, the number of drinks per drinking day, and the time to relapse to heavy drinking during a 12-week treatment trial. However, during a 14-week posttreatment follow-up period, study subjects showed a gradual increase in relapse rates, drinking days, and heavy drinking days, and the differences between naltrexone and placebo treatments no longer were statistically significant. In the COMBINE study, the advantage of naltrexone over placebo was retained after 16 weeks of treatment but diminished at 1-year follow-up (Anton et al., 2000). These findings suggest that patients may benefit from a longer duration of naltrexone treatment than the short-term therapies typically used in studies. However, the single major long-term treatment study published to date (Krystal et al., 2001) did not show a significant difference between naltrexone and placebo at 1-year follow-up.

Patient Selection The profile of a good candidate for oral naltrexone is based on an endophenotype of alcoholism consisting of a strong family history of alcoholism, euphoria or stimulation from alcohol, high levels of alcohol craving, and the presence of a variant of the mu-opioid receptor that results in greater sensitivity to beta-endorphin (O'Brien, 2006; Jaffe, Rounsaville et al., 1996). A retrospective analysis of genotypes in clinical trials of naltrexone indicate that the $A_{118}G$ allele, which codes for a mu receptor with increased sensitivity to b-endorphin, influences the treatment response to alcohol.

In a population study, the risk of developing alcoholism was increased in those who carry this allele. In another human laboratory study, the euphoric effects of alcohol in subjects of this genotype were enhanced compared to those with other alleles of the mu receptor gene.

In clinical trials, alcoholics with the gene for the sensitive form of the mu receptor did poorly when randomized to placebo but exceptionally well when randomized to naltrexone. A prospective study is in progress to determine whether treatment response to naltrexone among alcoholics can be predicted according to genotype. (Also see the discussion of the extended-release injectable formulation.)

Cautions and Contraindications Naltrexone is contraindicated in patients receiving long-term opioid therapy or opioid maintenance treatment because it could precipitate a severe opioid withdrawal syndrome. Naltrexone also is contraindicated in patients with hepatitis or liver failure (Doering, 1999).

Naltrexone has been shown to have dose-related hepatotoxicity, although generally this occurs at doses higher than those recommended for treatment of alcohol dependence. All patients should have hepatic transaminase levels checked regularly (Doering, 1999).

Use in Pregnancy Naltrexone is classified in FDA pregnancy category C (adverse effects on the fetus in animal studies, but no human trials have been conducted).

Use in Patients with Co-Occurring Medical or Psychiatric Disorders Naltrexone should not be used in patients undergoing long-term opioid therapy for chronic pain because of the risk of precipitating a severe withdrawal syndrome. It also should not be used in patients with hepatitis or liver failure (Doering, 1999). No other compatibility problems have been demonstrated with other psychiatric medications.

Clinical Recommendation Based on the weight of evidence for its effectiveness, oral naltrexone is recommended as an FDA-approved pharmacotherapy for the treatment of alcohol dependence in appropriately selected patients and in conjunction with psychosocial therapies (NIAAA, 2008).

Naltrexone (Extended-release Injectable Formulation)

A major improvement in the use of naltrexone is the availability of an extended release, injectable preparation that is active for 30 to 40 days. This greatly improves adherence and also reduces side effects, as well as minimizing the number of opportunities for patients to impulsively discontinue their medication (NIAAA, 2008). The extended-release formulation also affords the benefit of producing a more consistent and predictable blood level of the drug, since a depot injection bypasses first-pass metabolism (Johnson, 2007). As noted previously, naltrexone is an opioid antagonist with no intrinsic agonist properties.

Formulation and Dose The extended-release injectable formulation of naltrexone (Vivitrol®) is supplied as a microsphere formulation of naltrexone for suspension. It is administered once a month by intramuscular injection. (Also see the discussion of oral naltrexone.)

Mechanism of Action Naltrexone is believed to work by blocking mu-opioid receptors, thereby reducing the reinforcing effects of alcohol and leading to decreased feelings of intoxication and fewer cravings (Johnson, 2007).

Safety The extended-release injectable formulation of naltrexone generally is safe and well tolerated (Johnson, 2007). Reported adverse events are mild to moderate and typically resolved without intervention. The most common adverse events (nausea, headache, and injection site reactions) occurred at a rate similar to that for placebo (Johnson et al., 2003). (Also see the discussion of oral naltrexone in the preceding section). There is an FDA Black Box warning about liver damage when given in excessive doses.

Naltrexone does have the potential to interact with opioids and to precipitate severe withdrawal.

Efficacy In a 6-month, randomized, double-blind, placebo-controlled trial involving 624 individuals, 380 mg of long-acting naltrexone resulted in a 25% reduction in heavy drinking days compared to placebo, whereas a 190-mg dose resulted in a 17% reduction. The effect was larger in males (Garbutt et al., 2005).

One factor that appears to be important to naltrexone's effectiveness is adherence. For example, two studies found that oral naltrexone was effective only in the population of patients who were highly compliant with their medication regimen. However, alcoholics have been shown to have generally low rates of medication adherence. Nonadherence poses the additional problem that, if a patient on naltrexone wants to resume drinking or using drugs, he or she can readily discontinue the medication and experience the full effect of the drug. For these reasons, a sustained-release formulation would appear to be highly advantageous (Pettinati, Volpicelli et al., 2000b).

Patient Selection See the discussion of oral naltrexone.

Cautions and Contraindications Long-term opioid therapy (for chronic pain or substitution therapy for opioid dependence) is contraindicated because the naltrexone could precipitate a severe opioid withdrawal syndrome. Naltrexone also is contraindicated in patients with hepatitis or liver failure (Doering, 1999).

Naltrexone has been shown to have dose-related hepatotoxicity, although generally this occurs at doses higher than those recommended for treatment of alcohol dependence. All patients should have hepatic transaminase levels checked regularly (Doering, 1999).

Use in Pregnancy Naltrexone is classified in FDA pregnancy category C (adverse effects on the fetus in animal studies, but no human trials have been conducted).

Use in Patients with Co-Occurring Medical or Psychiatric Disorders Naltrexone should not be used in patients undergoing long-term opioid therapy for chronic pain because of the risk of precipitating a severe withdrawal syndrome. It also should not be used in patients with hepatitis or liver failure (Doering, 1999). No other compatibility problems have been demonstrated with other psychiatric medications.

Clinical Recommendation Based on the weight of evidence for its effectiveness, extended-release injectable (depot) naltrexone is recommended as an FDA-approved pharmacotherapy for the treatment of alcohol dependence in appropriately selected patients and in conjunction with psychosocial therapies (NIAAA, 2008).

EMERGING AND EXPERIMENTAL PHARMACOTHERAPIES

Although many patients have benefited from existing medications for the treatment of alcohol dependence, some fail to respond to them. Thus, a host of additional agents are under investigation.

Nalmefene

Nalmefene (Revex®), an opioid antagonist, is pharmacologically similar to naltrexone but lacks FDA approval for use in the treatment of alcohol dependence (Williams, 2005).

Outside of research settings, nalmefene is available at present only in injectable form, limiting its clinical utility (Williams, 2005).

Efficacy A pilot study in a small sample of alcoholics (Mason et al., 1994) showed an advantage for nalmefene 40 mg/day over nalmefene 10 mg/day or placebo in the prevention of relapse to heavy drinking. (Patients receiving nalmefene had a 37% relapse rate, compared with 59% in the placebo group [NNT = 5].) However, in a subsequent study by the same group, no difference was found between nalmefene 20 mg/day or 80 mg/day (Mason, Salvato, Williams, Ritvo, & Cutler, 1999).

Ondansetron

Ondansetron (Zofran®), a serotonin 5-HT3 antagonist, is not available for prescription as an oral medication, although it does have FDA approval for the treatment of nausea and is clinically available by the parenteral route (O'Brien, 2005).

Efficacy In a randomized controlled trial with a special oral formulation for research in alcoholics, investigators found a significant reduction in drinking among early-onset alcoholics. Specifically, at a dose substantially lower than that used to exert the antiemetic effects for which the medication is approved, ondansetron was superior to placebo in the proportion of abstinent days and the intensity of alcohol intake (Johnson et al., 2000). The early-onset alcoholic subtype is thought to have greater involvement of the serotonergic system, with a higher probability of antisocial behavior. (Among late-onset alcoholics, the effects of ondansetron on drinking behavior were, in nearly all respects, comparable to those of placebo [O'Brien, 2005].)

Ondansetron has been shown to yield favorable outcomes in patients with comorbid depression and alcohol dependence, particularly when combined with naltrexone (Dongier, 2005).

Based on the weight of evidence for its effectiveness, ondansetron is considered a promising pharmacotherapy to reduce drinking frequency and increase abstinence in appropriately selected patients and in conjunction with psychosocial therapies (Johnson et al., 2000, 2003; O'Brien, 2006).

Selective Serotonin Reuptake Inhibitors

Research into the use of selective serotonin reuptake inhibitors (SSRIs) to treat patients with alcohol dependence has been under way for the past decade, but most of the studies have used small samples and inconsistent outcome measures. Among the SSRIs tested in humans are zimelidine (Amit et al., 1985; Naranjo et al., 1984), fluvoxamine (Angelone, Bellini, Di Bella, & Catalano, 1998; Kranzler, Del Boca, Korner, & Brown, 1993), viqualine (Naranjo et al., 1989), sertraline (Pettinati, Volpicelli et al., 2000b), citalopram (Balldin et al., 1994; Naranjo et al., 1987; Naranjo, Poulos, Bremner, & Lanctot, 1992; Naranjo, Bremner, & Lanctot, 1995; Tiihonen, Ryynanen, Hakola, & Salaspuro, 1996), and fluoxetine (Gerra, Caccavari, Delsignore, & Bocchi,

1992; Gorelick & Paredes, 1992; Kabel & Petty, 1996; Kranzler et al., 1995; Naranjo, Kadlec, Sanhueza, Woodley-Remus, & Sellers, 1990). In the paragraphs that follow, the focus is on the two most intensively studied SSRIs: fluoxetine and citalopram.

Efficacy Studies suggest that SSRIs are efficacious only in heavy drinkers or in certain subgroups of patients. For example, Gerra and colleagues (1992) found an effect of fluoxetine only in alcoholics who had a positive family history of alcoholism. Balldin and colleagues (1994) found an effect of citalopram only among the heavier drinkers in their patient sample. By using a different approach to subtyping alcoholism, Kranzler, Burleson, Brown, and Babor (1996) found that high-risk/severity (Type B) alcoholism (one characteristic of which is an earlier age of onset) showed a poorer response to fluoxetine than to placebo. Prospective studies that aim to match SSRI treatment with alcoholic subtypes (based either on age of onset or a more complex subtyping procedure) may define a clearer role for such medications in the treatment of heavy drinking or alcohol dependence.

The emerging current consensus is that SSRIs may have a central role in depressed alcoholics, especially those with major depressive disorder; however, there is not yet enough clear evidence to warrant their use as first line therapies for alcoholism.

Topiramate

Although topiramate (Topamax®) has been approved by the FDA only for seizure disorders, preliminary clinical trials suggests that this GABAergic medication may significantly reduce drinking in alcoholics (NIAAA, 2008). The precise mechanism of action is unclear, but topiramate is thought to work by increasing inhibitory (GABA) neurotransmission and reducing stimulatory (glutamate) neurotransmission. It is available in oral form and requires a slow upward titration of dose to minimize side effects.

Efficacy In two randomized controlled trials, topiramate has been shown to significantly improve multiple drinking outcomes, compared with placebo (Johnson et al., 2003; Johnson et al., 2007). Over the course of a 14-week trial, topiramate significantly increased the proportion of volunteers with 28 consecutive days of abstinence or nonheavy drinking (Johnson et al., 2007). In both studies, the differences between topiramate and placebo groups were still diverging at the end of the trial, suggesting that the maximum effect may not have been reached. The magnitude of topiramate's effect may be larger than that for naltrexone or acamprosate. Importantly, efficacy was established in volunteers who were drinking at the time of starting the medication (Johnson, 2008; NIAAA, 2008).

Hypersensitivity to the drug is the only known contraindication. Adverse effects may include dizziness and somnolence (which are not dose-related), ataxia, impaired concentration, fatigue, paresthesias, speech difficulties, changes in sense of taste, diplopia, nausea, and decreased appetite. Interactions exist between topiramate and other anticonvulsants, including phenytoin (Dilantin®), valproic acid (Depakote®, Depakene®), and carbamazepine (Tegretol®).

Emerging consensus considers topiramate a second line agent at present, perhaps worthy of additional consideration in patients with bipolar disorder, as there is some evidence for moderate mood stabilizing effects as well (Johnson et al., 2000; Johnson, et al., 2003; NIAAA, 2008; O'Brien, 2005).

Summary

Critical barriers must be overcome to ensure that future efforts in the development of medications for alcohol use disorders reach full fruition. These challenges include establishing key targets for drug discovery, validating animal and human screening models, and developing biomarkers to help predict treatment success (Litten, Fertig, Mattson, & Egli, 2005; O'Brien, 2006).

In addition, it is important to formulate methodological and statistical strategies to efficiently conduct trials of alcohol pharmacotherapies; to specify genetic and phenotypic patient characteristics associated with efficacy and safety for lead compounds; to forge productive alliances among governmental agencies, the pharmaceutical industry, and academic researchers to further drug development; and, ultimately and perhaps most difficult, to engage the practitioner community to incorporate newly approved medications into their clinical practices (Litten et al., 2005).

CONSIDERATIONS IN DEVELOPING A TREATMENT PLAN

Offering a full range of effective treatment modalities maximizes patient choice and improves outcomes, as no single approach is universally successful or appealing to patients. The different approaches (medications for alcohol dependence, professional counseling, and mutual help groups) are complementary. They share the same goals while addressing different aspects of alcohol dependence: neurobiological, psychological, and social (NIAAA, 2008).

Selecting a Pharmacologic Agent

In general, when a pharmacologic therapy is indicated, the following factors should be considered in selecting a particular agent:

1. If a particular medication was helpful or effective in the past, then a repeat trial of the same medication should be considered. Alternatively, if a particular medication was not helpful or effective in an earlier trial, then the use of a different medication is warranted (ideally in combination with strategies to enhance adherence/compliance). The following factors should be considered in selecting a particular pharmacologic agent.
2. If the patient is actively drinking (less than 3 to 4 days of abstinence), consider oral naltrexone.
3. If the patient is not motivated for abstinence, (a) consider naltrexone or long-acting naltrexone in combination with motivational enhancement strategies; and (b) consider setting goals in consultation with the patient for a reduction in the frequency and amount of drinking (consider this as an interim motivational goal, with the expectation of moving toward abstinence as the ultimate goal).
4. If the risk of relapse is related to the patient's reports of subjective reward or pleasure associated with drinking (positive reinforcement), consider naltrexone or long-acting naltrexone.
5. If the risk of relapse is related to the patient's reports of relief of discomfort or dysphoria associated with drinking (negative reinforcement), consider acamprosate.
6. If the patient reports strong subjective cravings for alcohol, consider naltrexone or long-acting naltrexone.
7. If the patient has a strong family history of alcoholism, consider naltrexone or long-acting naltrexone.

8. If the patient is likely to have difficulty adhering to a medication regimen, consider long-acting injectable naltrexone.
9. If the patient also is addicted to opioids, consider long-acting injectable naltrexone (following withdrawal from the opioid) as therapy for both the alcohol and opioid dependence.
10. If the patient also is addicted to cocaine, consider disulfiram in combination with appropriate adherence enhancement measures.
11. If the patient is no more than moderately impulsive; is likely to be deterred by the imposition of tangible, immediate, and adverse consequences of drinking; and is committed to abstinence, consider disulfiram.
12. If the consequences of drinking involve imminent danger, consider disulfiram in combination with appropriate adherence enhancement measures.

A patient's willingness to abstain has important implications for the choice of medication. Most studies on effectiveness have required patients to abstain before starting treatment. A notable exception is topiramate, which was prescribed to study volunteers who were still drinking (Johnson et al., 2007).

Both oral and extended-release injection naltrexone may be helpful in reducing heavy drinking and encouraging abstinence in patients who are still drinking. However, its efficacy is much higher in patients who can abstain for 4 to 7 days before initiating treatment (Garbutt et al., 2005; Kranzler et al., 2003).

Acamprosate is approved only for use in patients who are abstinent at the start of treatment, and patients should be fully withdrawn before starting (NIAAA, 2008). Disulfiram is contraindicated in patients who wish to continue to drink, because a disulfiram–alcohol reaction occurs with any alcohol intake at all (NIAAA, 2008).

Contraindications and Cautions

The following factors either rule out the use of particular pharmacotherapies or indicate the need for special caution in their use.

1. Naltrexone is contraindicated in liver failure or acute hepatitis. In a patient with active liver disease (elevation of liver enzymes in the range of 4 to 5 times normal), the risk of naltrexone hepatotoxicity should be carefully considered and balanced against the hepatotoxicity of alcohol.
2. Acamprosate dose should be adjusted in the presence of renal insufficiency.
3. Disulfiram is contraindicated in the presence of severe cardiovascular disease, or severe hepatic or renal insufficiency or psychosis.
4. If injection is likely to be a barrier to acceptance, consider avoiding long-term injectable naltrexone.
5. If abstinence is unlikely because of the patient's severe impulsivity or a subjective intention to continue drinking, avoid disulfiram.

Specific medical factors that may influence the choice of medication are shown in Table 5-1.

Ultimately, the medication selected depends on the prescriber's clinical judgment and the patient's preference. Each drug has a different mechanism of action. Some patients may respond better to one medication than another (NIAAA, 2008). See Table 5-2.

TABLE 5-1

Summary: Medical Considerations in Selecting a Pharmacotherapy

	Oral Naltrexone (see pages 64–67)	*Extended-Release Injectable Naltrexone (see pages 67–68)*	*Acamprosate (see pages 60–62)*	*Disulfiram (see pages 62–64)*
Bleeding/Other Coagulation Disorders	A	C	A	A
Chronic Pain	C	C	A	A
Cognitive Impairment	A	A	A	X
Diabetes	A	A	A	C
Obesity that Precludes Intramuscular Injection	A	X	A	A
Psychosis	A	A	A	C
Renal Failure	A	A	X	A
Significant Liver Disease	C	C	A	C

A, appropriate to use; C, use with caution; X, contraindicated.

Source: Adapted from Center for Substance Abuse Treatment. (2009). *Tip 49: incorporating alcohol pharmacotherapies into medical practice*. Treatment Improvement Protocol (TIP) Series 49. HHS Publication No. (SMA) 09-4380. Rockville, MD: Substance Abuse and Mental Health Services Administration. Available online at: http://ncadistore.samhsa.gov/catalog/productDetails.aspx?ProductID=18117. Accessed December 1, 2009.

Combining Pharmacotherapies

A large U.S. trial found no benefit to combining acamprosate and naltrexone (Anton et al., 2006). Naltrexone, disulfiram, and both in combination were compared with placebo in the treatment of alcohol dependence in patients with coexisting Axis I psychiatric disorders (Petrakis et al., 2006). Equivalently better outcomes were obtained with either medication, but combining them did not have any additional effect. At this time, there is no evidence supporting the combination of medications, but the number of studies examining the question is limited.

Integration of Pharmacologic and Psychosocial Therapies

Almost all studies of medications for alcohol dependence have included some type of counseling, and support a recommendation that all patients receive at least brief counseling (Ernst, Pettinati, Weiss, Donovan, & Longabaugh, 2008). Evidence is accumulating that weekly or biweekly brief (i.e., 15–20 minutes) counseling by a health professional, combined with medication, is an effective treatment for many patients during early recovery (Anton et al., 2006; Johnson et al., 2007;

TABLE 5-2

Summary: Medications for Treating Alcohol Dependence

	Oral Naltrexone (see pages 64–67)	*Extended-Release Injectable Naltrexone (see pages 67–68)*	*Acamprosate (see pages 60–62)*	*Disulfiram (see pages 62–64)*	*Topiramate (see page 70)*
Actions	Blocks opioid receptors, resulting in reduced craving and reduced reward in response to drinking.	Same as oral naltrexone; 30-day duration	Affects glutamate and GABA neurotransmitter systems, but its overall mechanism of action is unclear.	Inhibits intermediate metabolism of alcohol, causing a build-up of acetaldehyde and a reaction of flushing, sweating, nausea, and tachycardia if a patient drinks alcohol.	Thought to work by increasing inhibitory (GABA) neurotransmission and reducing stimulatory (glutamate) neurotransmission.
Indications *Adherence should be considered as a potential limitation to the effectiveness of all medications.*	If the patient reports (1) subjective reward or pleasure from drinking (positive reinforcement); (2) strong subjective cravings for alcohol; (3) a strong positive family history of alcoholism; or (4) a lack of motivation toward abstinence.	Same as oral naltrexone, or if the patient reports that adherence to oral naltrexone is a problem or the patient is dependent on an opioid drug (following opioid withdrawal).	If the patient reports (1) relief of dysphoria or discomfort from drinking (negative reinforcement); (2) an extensive history of withdrawal symptoms; (3) anxiety or apprehension about withdrawal; or (4) a significant protracted abstinence syndrome.	If the consequences of drinking are imminently dangerous and/or potentially devastating, and if coupled with suitable adherence enhancement measures, particularly monitored medication administration. If the patient reports: (1) a goal of abstinence and moderate impulsivity; (2) if the patient also is dependent on cocaine.	If the patient has a history of poorly controlled bipolar disorder, consider topiramate, which may have the additional benefit of augmenting a primary mood-stabilizing medication in addition to its potential benefit for alcohol dependence (although it is not FDA-approved for either of these indications).
Contra-indications	Also using opioids or in acute opioid withdrawal; anticipated need to administer	Same as oral naltrexone. Also, inadequate muscle mass for deep in-	Severe renal impairment (CrCI ≤30 mL/min)	Concomitant use of alcohol or alcohol-containing preparations or metronidazole; coronary artery	Hypersensitivity to topiramate

	opioids for pain; acute hepatitis or liver failure.	tramuscular injection, or rash or infection at the injection site.		disease; severe myocardial disease; hypersensitivity to rubber derivatives (thiuram).	
Precautions *Advise patients to carry a wallet card to alert medical personnel in the event of emergency (see http://www.niaaa.nih.gov/guide)*	Other hepatic disease; renal impairment; history of suicide attempts or depression. If opioid analgesia is needed, larger doses may be required and respiratory depression may be deeper and more prolonged. Pregnancy Category C.	Same as oral naltrexone, in addition to hemophilia or other bleeding problems	Moderate renal impairment (dose adjustment for CrCI between 30 and 50 mL/min); depression or suicidal ideation or behavior. Pregnancy Category C.	Hepatic cirrhosis or insufficiency; cerebrovascular disease or cerebral damage; psychoses (past or present); diabetes mellitus; epilepsy; hypothyroidism; renal impairment. Pregnancy Category C.	Narrow angle glaucoma; kidney stones; renal or hepatic impairment; severely underweight; use of central nervous system depression. Pregnancy Category C.
Serious Adverse Reactions	Will precipitate severe withdrawal if the patient is dependent on opioids; hepatotoxicity (although it does not appear to be a hepatotoxin at the recommended doses)	Hepatotoxicity (although it does not appear to be a hepatotoxin at the recommended doses); injection site reactions that may be severe (instruct patients to closely monitor site and seek care immediately if reaction is worsening). Also, depression and rare	Rare events include suicidal ideation and behavior.	Disulfiram-alcohol interaction; hepatotoxicity; optic neuritis; peripheral neuropathy; psychotic reactions	Metabolic acidosis; acute myopia and secondary narrow-angle glaucoma; oligohidrosis and hyperthermia

(continues)

TABLE 5-2

Summary: Medications for Treating Alcohol Dependence *(continued)*

	Oral Naltrexone (see pages 64–67)	*Extended-Release Injectable Naltrexone (see pages 67–68)*	*Acamprosate (see pages 60–62)*	*Disulfiram (see pages 62–64)*	*Topiramate (see page 70)*
		events that may include allergic pneumonia and suicidal ideation or behavior.			
Common Side Effects	Nausea, vomiting, decreased appetite; headache; dizziness; fatigue; anxiety	Same as oral naltrexone, plus a reaction at the injection site; joint pain; muscle aches or cramps	Diarrhea; somnolence	Metallic after-taste; dermatitis; transient mild drowsiness	Paresthesias; taste perversion; anorexia and weight loss; somnolence; cognitive dysfunction
Interactions With Other Drugs	Opioid medications (blocks actions)	Same as oral naltrexone	No clinically relevant interactions reported.	Anticoagulants such as warfarin, isoniazid, metronidazole, phenytoin; any over-the-counter agent containing alcohol	Other anticonvulsants; other carbonic anhydrase inhibitors; hydrochlorothiazide; metformin; pioglitazone; lithium; amitriptylene
Usual Adult Dose	***Oral dose:*** 50–100 mg, given daily. ***Before prescribing:*** Patients must be opioid-free for a minimum of	***Intramuscular dose:*** 380 mg, given as a deep intramuscular gluteal injection,	***Oral dose:*** 666 mg (two 333 mg tablets), given three times a day. For patients with moderate renal impairment	***Oral dose:*** 250 mg (with a range of 125 mg to 500 mg), given daily. ***Before prescribing:*** Evaluate liver function. Warn the	***Oral dose:*** Initially, 25 mg at bedtime, increased each week by 25 mg to 50 mg a day, divided into morning and

	7 to 10 days before starting medication. If an opioid withdrawal reaction is a possibility, a naloxone challenge test should be administered before naltrexone is given. Evaluate liver function. ***Laboratory follow-up:*** Monitor liver function	once a month ***Before prescribing:*** Same as oral naltrexone. Also, examine the injection site for adequate muscle mass and skin condition. ***Laboratory follow-up:*** Monitor liver function	(CrCI 30 to 50 mL/min), reduce to 333 mg (one tablet) three times a day. ***Before prescribing:*** Evaluate renal function; establish abstinence	patient (1) not to take disulfiram for at least 12 hours after drinking, and that a disulfiram-ethanol reaction can occur up to 2 weeks after the last dose; and (2) to avoid alcohol in food (e.g., sauces, vinegars), over-the-counter medications (cough syrups), and toiletries (cologne, mouthwash). ***Laboratory follow-up:*** Monitor liver function	evening doses (faster titration is likely to cause adverse reactions). Target dose is 200 mg per day, but patients unable to tolerate that dose may respond to lower doses. ***Before prescribing:*** Evaluate renal function, obtain serum electrolytes and bicarbonate. ***Laboratory follow-up:*** Monitor renal function, serum electrolytes, and bicarbonate.

Note: This chart highlights some of the properties of each medication, but it does not provide complete information and is not intended as a substitute for the package inserts or other reference sources used by clinicians. For patient information about these and other drugs, the National Library of Medicine operates MedlinePlus (http://medlineplus.gov). Whether or not a medication should be prescribed and in what amounts is a matter to be determined by the treating physician in response to the situation of each individual patient. Also note that while topiramate may be prescribed "off label," it is not yet approved by the Food and Drug Administration for the treatment of alcohol dependence. *Source:* Adapted from National Institute on Alcohol Abuse and Alcoholism. (2008). *Helping patients who drink too much: A clinician's guide.* Bethesda, MD: NIAAA, National Institutes of Health. Available online at: http://www.niaaa.nih.gov/Publications/EducationTrainingMaterials/guide.htm. Accessed September 17, 2009.

O'Malley, Rounsaville et al., 2003). Such counseling focuses on encouraging abstinence, adherence to the treatment regimen, and participation in support groups.

As with pharmacotherapies, the type of psychosocial intervention given is an important variable. As the research literature on the use of these drugs grows, it will be possible to assess their utility in conjunction with a variety of psychosocial therapies or as one element in a multimodal program for the treatment of alcohol use disorders. Advances in controlling the "dose" of psychosocial treatments through a manual-guided treatment approach promise to allow caregivers to optimize the ways in which particular medications are combined with specific psychosocial treatments (Johnson, 2008; Kranzler & Jaffe, 2003).

As with commitment to abstain, a patient's ability to adhere to the treatment regimen is a major consideration in deciding whether to use a pharmacotherapy, as well as in selecting a particular agent. Because less than optimal adherence to medication regimens is not the exception but the norm, the need for some level of adherence enhancement (such as motivational enhancement) should be considered part of standard treatment rather than a special procedure. Standard compliance/adherence enhancement strategies are listed in Table 5-3.

In addition to these standard measures, certain circumstances require more intensive adherence enhancement strategies, as shown in Table 5-4. For example, if medication adherence is a problem or assessed as likely to be a problem, one or more of these special enhancement strategies should be considered.

Attention to treatment adherence is the responsibility of the entire treatment team. While physicians traditionally have taken the lead in monitoring medication use and encouraging adherence to the therapeutic regimen, nonprescribers also have an essential role in successfully integrating pharmacologic and psychosocial treatments and thereby optimizing patient outcomes.

When medication management and addiction treatment services are being delivered by separate providers, close coordination and integration of services is required. Addiction treatment staff and addiction medicine physicians who have special training and experience in evaluating patients and prescribing pharmacotherapies for alcoholism and/or co-occurring medical or psychiatric disorders should develop close linkages with one another.

TABLE 5-3

Standard Strategies to Enhance Medication Compliance/Adherence

1. Monitoring by the health care team, including explicit inquiries (through nonjudgmental questions) to obtain an accurate medication use history;
2. Coordination and collaboration between the medical and counseling staff around medication monitoring;
3. Encouragement and monitoring by the counselor or therapist; and
4. Role induction to establish and reinforce medication adherence. As in all treatment, the earlier the role is induced, the more likely the patient is to incorporate medication-taking into his or her daily routine.

TABLE 5-4

Special Strategies to Enhance Medication Compliance/Adherence

- Intensified medication monitoring by the health care team, involving increased intensity or frequency of monitoring by the medical staff and, perhaps, the use of standardized questionnaires.
- Increased coordination and collaboration between the medical and counseling staffs around medication monitoring, possibly involving standardized protocols for communication.
- Encouragement and intensive monitoring of the patient by a counselor or therapist, possibly involving inclusion of medication adherence as a counseling treatment goal.
- Use of intensive manualized approaches, such as those from the Medication Management and BRENDA manuals from Project COMBINE.
- Use of *network therapy* (engagement of a concerned other in monitoring the patient's medication adherence) and notifying the prescriber about any problems observed.
- Supervision of medication self-administration or direct administration by a caregiver.
- Use of motivational incentives, contingency management, or other rewards for medication adherence.
- Use of a long-acting medication, such as extended-release injectable naltrexone.
- Use of a criminal justice mandate or other external forms of pressure (e.g., risk of loss of a primary relationship), if available.
- Intensification of the level of care to provide increased support, monitoring, and/or supervision.

Duration of Treatment

The risk for relapse to alcohol dependence is very high in the first 6 to 12 months after initiating abstinence and gradually diminishes over several years. Therefore, a minimum initial period of 3 months of pharmacotherapy is recommended.

Although an optimal treatment duration has not been established, it is reasonable to continue treatment for a year or longer if the patient responds to medication. After the medication is discontinued, patients may need to be followed more closely. Pharmacotherapy may be reinstated if relapse occurs (NIAAA, 2008).

MANAGEMENT OF CO-OCCURRING DISORDERS

Differential Diagnosis

Although many patients feel considerably better after their acute withdrawal symptoms abate, for others the anxiety, insomnia, and general distress of the acute withdrawal syndrome merge imperceptibly into a postwithdrawal state that can last for weeks or months. Some aspects of this postacute withdrawal (such as irritability or insomnia) are referred to as persistent abstinence effects or "protracted" or "subacute" withdrawal. Multiple factors contribute to this phenomenon, including (1) heavy alcohol intake; (2) acute and protracted withdrawal; (3) alcohol-induced damage to the central nervous system; (4) damage to the central nervous system from indirect effects of alcohol (e.g., head trauma or thiamine deficiency); (5) social, economic, and interpersonal losses; (6) antecedent psychiatric disorders; and (7) a cluster of signs and symptoms that may be referred to as the "defeat/depression/ hypophoria cluster" (Kranzler & Jaffe, 2003).

However, other symptoms may signal the emergence of diagnosable psychiatric disorders. The relationship between substance use and psychiatric symptomatology is complex (Kranzler & Rounsaville, 1998; Myers, Borg et al., 1986). Epidemiologic studies document high rates of comorbid psychiatric disorders in alcohol-dependent individuals in the community (Grant & Harford, 1995; Kessler et al., 1994; Kessler et al., 1997; Regier et al., 1990). In fact, most individuals who seek treatment for their alcohol dependence meet lifetime criteria for psychiatric disorders in addition to alcoholism. These disorders commonly include major depression, bipolar disorder, antisocial personality disorder, drug dependence, borderline personality disorder, phobias, and attention deficit/hyperactivity disorder (Behar & Winokur, 1979; Dongier, 2005; Hesselbrock & Meyer, 1985; Mullaney & Trippett, 1979; Nace, Saxon, & Shore, 1983; Ross, Glaser, & Germanson, 1988; Wood, Wender, & Reimherr, 1983).

Depressive symptoms and depressive disorders are among the most common to present comorbidly. Many persons who enter treatment for alcohol dependence have high scores on depression rating scales (as for example when measured in research studies), but these symptoms often decline after a few weeks of abstinence. However, even if one accepts the view that many of these psychiatric symptoms will remit spontaneously within a few days to several weeks (Brown & Schuckit, 1988; Schuckit, 1983), there are many patients whose severe and persistent symptoms will *not* remit spontaneously and instead require additional treatment (Williams, 2005). Additionally, untreated depression can increase the risk of relapse by contributing to impairments in motivational pathways underlying craving and reinforcement (Dongier, 2005).

In some cases where depressive symptoms are primary, an alcohol use disorder may have developed in the course of attempts at "self-medication." In other cases, the diagnosis of comorbid depression—as well as the treatment plan based on that diagnosis—must be reevaluated if it can be determined that the depressive symptoms are exclusively secondary to the alcohol dependence. In most cases, it may be impossible to determine precisely which disorder is primary, either chronologically or etiologically. More typically, the best we can do when comorbid depressive disorders are present is to understand them as mutually exacerbating and sustaining. Absent of the ability to precisely determine which disorder is primary, then both disorders should be considered primary and be provided with simultaneous, integrated treatment. Some of the important factors in making the diagnosis include: previous symptoms during periods of abstinence or reduced use, presence of full syndromal diagnostic criteria, previous treatment response, family history, chronological onset if determinable, chronicity, and severity.

Two symptoms of depressive disorders require special attention in relation to alcohol dependence. First, the risk of suicide among individuals with both conditions is higher than among persons who are depressed but not experiencing problems with alcohol. Suicide often is impulsive and facilitated by intoxication. Second, in depressed patients, insomnia may persist for months after they initiate abstinence and is a predictor of relapse (Dongier, 2005).

Psychosocial approaches for comorbid psychiatric disorders provided in conjunction with pharmacologic therapy include cognitive-behavioral therapy, which has proved effective for both depression and alcohol dependence, and motivational interviewing, which maximize the potential for improved long-term outcomes (Dongier, 2005).

Pharmacologic Therapies

Among the drugs that have been used or proposed to treat co-occurring psychiatric disorders are SSRI antidepressants (such as fluoxetine or citalopram), tricyclic antidepressants (e.g., imipramine or desipramine), benzodiazepines and other anxiolytics, antipsychotics (e.g., phenothiazines and other dopaminergic blockers), and mood stabilizing agents (e.g., lithium). The use of these drugs in alcoholics requires careful consideration of the potential for adverse effects in this patient population, which may be attributable to co-occurring medical disorders (often present among alcoholics). The pharmacokinetic effects of acute and chronic alcohol consumption are also important. For example, it has been shown that chronic ethanol administration increases clearance of imipramine and desipramine, potentially reducing the effectiveness of these medications (Ciraulo et al., 1982; Ciraulo, Barnhill et al., 1988). Further, disulfiram can interact with these and other medications used to treat comorbid psychiatric disorders (Ciraulo et al., 1985; Gorelick, 1993).

While it is critical to attempt to treat the pathologic mood states that may be important in the initiation and sustaining of heavy drinking, it also is important to note that medications that ameliorate persistent mood symptoms will not necessarily by themselves produce changes in alcohol consumption once a significant degree of alcohol dependence develops. Once the neuroadaptive changes and the complex learning that constitute the dependence syndrome occur, alcohol dependence becomes autonomous, and often does not resolve simply because one major contributing factor is brought under control (Edwards & Gross, 1976; Wikler, 1980). Pharmacological treatment of comorbid psychiatric disorders must therefore be part of a broader treatment strategy that includes interventions that specifically target alcohol dependence.

Contraindications and Cautions

The presence of a co-occurring psychiatric disorder requires special care in the use of pharmacotherapies.

- Both naltrexone and acamprosate may be used in combination with psychiatric medications, as there are no known drug interactions between these classes of medication.
- If the patient exhibits chronic psychiatric symptoms (e.g., depression, mood lability, psychosis, anxiety, etc.), consider the "self-medication" hypothesis and possible concurrent pharmacologic treatment for potential psychiatric comorbidity.
- If the patient has a history of poorly controlled bipolar disorder, consider topiramate, which may have the additional benefit of augmenting a primary mood stabilizing medication in addition to its potential benefit for alcohol dependence (*note that this indication is not approved by the FDA*).
- If the patient exhibits symptoms of chronic depression, consider an antidepressant (unless there is a history of mania or hypomania).
- Disulfiram is contraindicated by the presence of psychosis because of the risk that it will exacerbate the psychotic symptoms.
- Disulfiram may increase blood levels and hence the effects of tricyclic antidepressants and long-acting hepatically metabolized benzodiazepines.

REFERENCES

Agency for Health Care Policy and Research. (1999). *Pharmacotherapy for Alcohol Dependence* [Summary, Evidence Report/Technology Assessment Number 3]. Rockville, MD: AHRQ, U.S. Department of Health and Human Services.

Alford, D. P. (2003). Surgical interventions in the alcohol- or drug-using patient. In A. W. Graham, T. K. Schultz, M. F. Mayo-Smith, R. K. Ries, & B. B. Wilford (Eds.), *Principles of addiction medicine.* (3rd ed.). Chevy Chase, MD: American Society of Addiction Medicine.

Allen, J. P., & Litten, R. Z. (1992). Techniques to enhance compliance with disulfiram. *Alcoholism: Clinical & Experimental Research, 16,* 1035–1041.

Al-Otaiba, Z., Worden, B. L., McCrady, B. S., & Epstein, E. E. (2008). Accounting for self-selected drinking goals in the assessment of treatment outcome. *Psychology of Addictive Behaviors, 22,* 3, 439–443.

Altun, G., Altun, A., & Erdogan, O. (2007). Acute myocardial infarction due to disulfiram-alcohol interaction. *Cardiovascular Drugs and Therapy, 20,* 5, 391–392.

Amit, Z., Brown, Z., Sutherland, A., Rockman, G., Gill, K., & Selvaggi, N. (1985). Reduction in alcohol intake in humans as a function of treatment with zimelidine: Implications for treatment. In: C. A. Naranjo, & E. M. Sellers (Eds.). *Research advances in new psychopharmacological treatments for alcoholism.* (pp. 189–198). Amsterdam, The Netherlands: Elsevier.

Angelone, S. M., Bellini, L., Di Bella, D., & Catalano, M. (1998). Effects of fluvoxamine and citalopram in maintaining abstinence in a sample of Italian detoxified alcoholics. *Alcohol and Alcoholism, 33,* 151–156.

Anton, R.F. (2008a). Genetic basis for predicting response to naltrexone in the treatment of alcohol dependence. *Pharmacogenomics, 9,* 6, 655–658.

Anton, R. F. (2008b). Naltrexone for the management of alcohol dependence. *New England Journal of Medicine, 359,* 7, 715–721.

Anton, R. F., Moak, D. H., Waid, R., Latham, P. K., Malcolm, R. J., & Dias, J. K. (1999). Naltrexone and cognitive behavioral therapy for the treatment of outpatient alcoholics: Results of a placebo-controlled trial. *American Journal of Psychiatry, 156,* 1758–1764.

Anton, R. F., Moak, D. H., Latham, P. K., Waid, L. R., Malcolm, R. J., Dias, J. K, et al. (2000). Post-treatment results of combining naltrexone and cognitive-behavior therapy for the treatment of alcoholism. *Journal of Clinical Psychopharmacology, 21,* 72–77.

Anton, R. F., O'Malley, S. S., Ciraulo, D. A., Cisler, R. A., Couper, D., Donovan, D. M., et al. (2006). Combined pharmacotherapies and behavioral interventions for alcohol dependence: the COMBINE study: A randomized controlled trial. *Journal of the American Medical Association, 295,* 17, 2003–2017.

Azrin, N. H., Sisson, R. W., Meyers, R., & Godley, M. (1982). Alcoholism treatment by disulfiram and community reinforcement therapy. *Journal of Behavior Therapy and Experimental Psychiatry, 13,* 105–112.

Balldin, J., Berggren, U., Engel, J., Eriksson, M., Hard, E., & Soderpalm, B. (1994). Effect of citalopram on alcohol intake in heavy drinkers. *Alcoholism: Clinical & Experimental Research, 18,* 1133–1136.

Baros, A. M., Latham, P. K., & Anton, R. F. (2008). Naltrexone and cognitive behavioral therapy for the treatment of alcohol dependence: Do sex differences exist? *Alcoholism, Clinical and Experimental Research, 32,* 5, 771–776.

Batki, S. L., Meszaros, Z. S., Strutynski, K., Dimmock, J. A., Leontieva, L., Ploutz-Snyder, R., et al. (2008). Medical comorbidity in patients with schizophrenia and alcohol dependence. *Schizophrenia Research, 107,* 139–146.

Behar, D., & Winokur, G. (1979). Research in alcoholism and depression: A two-way street under construction. In: R. W. Pickens, & L. L. Heston (Eds.). *Psychiatric factors in drug abuse.* (pp. 125–152). New York: Grune & Stratton.

Bliding, A. (1978). The abuse potential of benzodiazepines with special reference to oxazepam. *Acta Psychiatrica Scandinavica,* (Suppl 24), 111–116.

Brown, S. A., & Schuckit, M. A. (1988). Changes in depression among abstinent alcoholics. *Journal of Studies on Alcohol, 49,* 412–417.

Bergstrom, B., Ohlin, H., Lindblom, P. E., & Wadstein, J. (1982). Is disulfiram implantation effective? *Lancet, 1,* 49–50.

Besson, J., Aeby, F., Kasas, A., Lehert, P., & Potgieter, A. (1998). Combined efficacy of acamprosate and disulfiram in the treatment of alcoholism: A controlled study. *Alcoholism: Clinical & Experimental Research, 22,* 573–579.

Blanc, M., & Daeppen, J. B. (2005). Does disulfiram still have a role in alcoholism treatment? *Revue Medicale Suisse, 1*, 26, 1728–1730, 1732–1733.

Boothby, L. A., & Doering, P. L. (2005). Acamprosate for the treatment of alcohol dependence. *Clinical Therapeutics, 27*, 6, 695–714.

Bouza, C., Angeles, M., Muñoz, A., & Amate, J. M. (2004). Efficacy and safety of naltrexone and acamprosate in the treatment of alcohol dependence: A systematic review. *Addiction, 99*, 7, 811–828.

Brady, K. T., Myrick, H., Henderson, S., & Coffey, S. F. (2002). The use of divalproex in alcohol relapse prevention: A pilot study. *Drug and Alcohol Dependence, 67*, 323–330.

Brewer, C., Meyers, R. J., & Johnsen, J. (2000). Does disulfiram help to prevent relapse in alcohol abuse? *CNS Drugs, 14*, 329–341.

Buonopane, A., & Petrakis, I. L. (2005). Pharmacotherapy of alcohol use disorders. *Substance Use & Misuse, 40*, 2001–2020, 2043–2048.

Carroll, K. M., Rounsaville, B. J., & Gawin, F. H. (1991). A comparative trial of psychotherapies for ambulatory cocaine abusers: Relapse prevention and interpersonal psychotherapy. *American Journal of Drug and Alcohol Abuse, 17*, 229–247.

Carroll, K. M., & Schottenfeld, R. (1997). Nonpharmacologic approaches to substance abuse treatment. *The Medical Clinics of North America, 81*, 4, 927–944.

Catalano, R., Howard, M., Hawkins, J., et al. (1988). Relapse in the addictions: rates, determinants, and promising prevention strategies. *1988 Surgeon General's Report on health consequences of smoking*. Washington, DC: Office of Smoking and Health, Department of Health and Human Services.

Chatterjee, C. R., & Ringold, A. L. (1999). A case report of reduction in alcohol craving and protection against alcohol withdrawal by gabapentin. *Journal of Clinical Psychiatry, 60*, 617.

Chick, J. (1999). Safety issues concerning the use of disulfiram in treating alcohol dependence. *Drug Safety, 20*, 427–435.

Chick, J., Anton, R., Checinski, K., Croop, R., Drummond, D. C., Farmer, R., et al. (2000). A multicentre, randomized, double-blind, placebo-controlled trial of naltrexone in the treatment of alcohol dependence or abuse. *Alcohol and Alcoholism, 35*, 587–593.

Chick, J., Gough, K., Falkowski, W., Kershaw, P., Hore, B., Mehta, B., et al. (1992). Disulfiram treatment of alcoholism. *British Journal of Psychiatry, 161*, 84–89.

Ciraulo, D. A., Alderson, L. M., Chapron, D. J., Jaffe, J. H., Subbarao, B., & Kramer, P. A. (1982). Imipramine disposition in alcoholics. *Journal of Clinical Psychopharmacology, 2*, 2–7.

Ciraulo, D. A., Barnhill, J., & Boxenbaum, H. G. (1985). Pharmacokinetic interaction of disulfiram and antidepressants. *American Journal of Psychiatry, 142*, 1373–1374.

Ciraulo, D. A., Barnhill, J. G., Jaffe, J. H., Ciraulo, A. M., & Tarmey, M. F. (1990). Intravenous pharmacokinetics of 2-hydroxyimipramine in alcoholics and normal controls. *Journal of Studies on Alcohol, 51*, 366–372.

Ciraulo, D. A., Dong, Q., Silverman, B. L., Gastfriend, D. R., & Pettinati, H. M. (2008). Early treatment response in alcohol dependence with extended-release naltrexone. *Journal of Clinical Psychiatry, 69*, 2, 190–195.

Comer, S. D., Collins, E. D., Kleber, H. D., Nuwayser, E. S., Kerrigan, J. H., & Fischman, M. W. (2002). Depot naltrexone: Long-lasting antagonism of the effects of heroin in humans. *Psychopharmacology (Berl), 159*, 351–360.

Connors, G. J., Longabaugh, R., & Miller, W. R. (1996). Looking forward and back to relapse: implications for research and practice. *Addiction, 91*, Suppl., 191–196.

Cornelius, J. R., Salloum, I. M., Cornelius, M. D., Perel, J. M., Thase, M. E., Ehler, J. G., et al. (1993). Fluoxetine trial in suicidal depressed alcoholics. *Psychopharmacology Bulletin, 29*, 195–199.

Crits-Christoph, P. L., Siqueland, L., Blaine, J., Frank, A., Luborsky, L., Onken, L. S., et al. (1999). Psychosocial treatments for cocaine dependence: National Institute on Drug Abuse Collaborative Cocaine Treatment Study. *Archives of General Psychiatry, 56*, 493–502.

Croop, R. S., Faulkner, E. B., & Labriola, D. F. (1997). The safety profile of naltrexone in the treatment of alcoholism: Results from a multicenter usage study. *Archives of General Psychiatry, 54*, 1130–1135.

Daley, D. C. (2000). *Relapse prevention workbook for recovering alcoholics and drug dependent persons, 3rd edition.* Holmes Beach, FL: Learning Publications.

Daley, D. C., & Raskin, M. S. (1991). *Treating the chemically dependent and their families.* Newbury Park, CA: Sage Publications.

Daley, D. C., Salloum, I. M., Zuckoff, A., Kirisci, L., & Thase, M. E. (1998). Increasing treatment compliance among outpatients with depression and cocaine dependence: results of a pilot study. *American Journal of Psychiatry, 155*, 1611–1613.

Dawes, M. A., Johnson, B. A., Ma, J. Z., Ait-Daoud, N., Thomas, S. E., & Cornelius, J. R. (2005). Reductions in and relations between "craving" and drinking in a prospective, open-label trial of ondansetron in adolescents with alcohol dependence. *Addictive Behavior, 30*, 9, 1630–1637.

Delaney, H. D., Forcehimes, A. A., Campbell, W. P., & Smith, B. W. (2009). Integrating spirituality into alcohol treatment. *Journal of Clinical Psychology, 65*, 2, 185–198.

De Sousa, A. A., De Sousa, J., & Kapoor, H. (2008). An open randomized trial comparing disulfiram and topiramate in the treatment of alcohol dependence. *Journal of Substance Abuse Treatment, 34*, 4, 460–463.

De Witte, P., Littleton, J., Parot, P., & Koob, G. et al. (2005). Neuroprotective and abstinence-promoting effects of acamprosate: Elucidating the mechanism of action. *CNS Drugs, 19*, 6, 517–537.

Diehl, A., & Mann, K. (2007). Pharmacological relapse prevention in alcohol and tobacco dependence. *Internist (Berl), 48*, 1, 79–84, 86–88.

Dimeff, L. A., & Marlatt, G. A. (1995). Relapse prevention. In: R. Hester, & W. Miller. (Eds.) *Handbook of alcoholism treatment approaches. (2nd ed., pp. 176–194)*. Boston, MA: Allyn & Bacon.

Doering, P. L. (1999). Substance-related disorders: Alcohol, nicotine, and caffeine. In: J. T. DiPiro, R. L. Talbert, G. C. Yee, G. M. Matzke, B. Wells, & M. Posey. (Eds.). *Pharmacotherapy: A pathophysiologic approach.* (4th ed.). Stamford, CT: Appleton & Lange.

Dongier, M. (2005). Psychopharmacology for the clinician. *Reviews of Psychiatry and Neuroscience (Canada), 30*, 3.

Donovan, D. M., Anton, R. F., Miller, W. R., Longabaugh, R., Hosking, J. D., Youngblood, M., for the COMBINE Study Research Group. (2008). Combined pharmacotherapies and behavioral interventions for alcohol dependence (The COMBINE Study): Examination of posttreatment drinking outcomes. *Journal of Studies on Alcohol and Drugs, 69*, 1, 5–13.

Dorus, W., Ostrow, D. G., Anton, R., Cushman, P., Collins, J. F., Shaefer, M., et al. (1989). Lithium treatment of depressed and nondepressed alcoholics. *Journal of the American Medical Association*, 262, 1646–1652.

Drummond, D. C., Litten, R. Z., Lowman, C., & Hunt, W. A. (2000). Craving research: future directions. *Addiction, 95*, Suppl. 2, S247–255.

Dundon, W. D., Pettinati, H. M., Lynch, K. G., Xie, H., Varillo, K. M., Makadon, C., et al. (2008). The therapeutic alliance in medical-based interventions impacts outcome in treating alcohol dependence. *Drug and Alcohol Dependence, 95*, 3, 230–236.

Edwards, G., & Gross, M. M. (1976). Alcohol dependence: Provisional description of a clinical syndrome. *British Medical Journal, 1*, 1058–1061.

Ernst, D. B., Pettinati, H. M., Weiss, R. D., Donovan, D. M., & Longabaugh, R. (2008). An intervention for treating alcohol dependence: Relating elements of Medical Management to patient outcomes with implications for primary care. *Annals of Family Medicine, 6*, 5, 435–40.

Flórez, G., García-Portilla, P., Alvarez, S., Saiz, P. A., Nogueiras, L., & Bobes, J. (2008). Using topiramate or naltrexone for the treatment of alcohol-dependent patients. *Alcoholism, Clinical Experimental Research*, 32, 7, 1251–1259.

Fuller, R. K., Branchey, L., Brightwell, D. R., Derman, R. M., Emrick, C. D., Iber, F. L., et al. (1986). Disulfiram treatment of alcoholism. A Veterans Administration cooperation study. *Journal of the American Medical Association*, 256, 1449–1455.

Fuller, R. K., & Gordis, E. (2004). Does disulfiram have a role in alcoholism treatment today? *Addiction, 99*, 1, 21–24.

Galanter, M. (2008). The concept of spirituality in relation to addiction recovery and general psychiatry. *Recent Developments in Alcoholism*, 18, 125–140.

Garbutt, J. C. (2009). The state of pharmacotherapy for the treatment of alcohol dependence. *Journal of Substance Abuse Treatment, 36*, 1, S15–23.

Garbutt, J. C., Kranzler, H. R., O'Malley, S. S., Gastfriend, D. R., Pettinati, H. M, Silverman, B. L., et al. (2005). Efficacy and tolerability of long-acting injectable naltrexone for alcohol dependence: A randomized controlled trial. *Journal of the American Medical Association*, 293, 1617–1625.

Garbutt, J. C., West, S. L., Carey, T. S., Lohr, K. N., Crews, F. T., et al. (1999). Pharmacological treatment of alcohol dependence: A review of the evidence. *Journal of the American Medical Association, 281*, 1318–1325.

Gastfriend, D. R., Garbutt, J. C., Pettinati, H. M., & Forman, R. F. (2007). Reduction in heavy drinking as a treatment outcome in alcohol dependence. *Journal of Substance Abuse Treatment, 33*, 1, 71–80.

Geerlings, P. J., Ansoms, C., & van den Brink, W. (1997). Acamprosate and prevention of relapse in alcoholics. *European Addiction Research, 3*, 129–137.

Gerra, G., Caccavari, R., Delsignore, R., & Bocchi, R. (1992). Effects of fluoxetine and Ca-acetyl-homotaurinate on alcohol intake in familial and nonfamilial alcohol patients. *Current Therapeutic Research, 52*, 291–295.

Gianoulakis, C. (1990). Characterization of the effects of acute ethanol administration on the release of β-endorphin peptides by the rat hypothalamus. *European Journal of Pharmacology, 180*, 21–29.

Goldberg, H. L., & Finnerty, R. J. (1979). The comparative efficacy of buspirone and diazepam in the treatment of anxiety. *American Journal of Psychiatry, 136*, 1184–1187.

Goldberg, J. F., Garno, J. L., Leon, A. C., Kocsis, J. H., & Portera, L. (1999). A history of substance abuse complicates remission from acute mania in bipolar disorder. Journal of Clinical Psychiatry, 60, 733–740.

Goldstein, B., Diamantouros, A., Schaffer, A., & Naranjo, C. A. (2006). Pharmacotherapy of alcoholism in patients with co-morbid psychiatric disorders. Review article. *Drugs, 66*, 9, 1229–1237.

Gorelick, D. A. (1993). Recent developments in pharmacological treatment of alcoholism. In: M. Galanter. (Ed.). *Recent developments in alcoholism, Vol. 11.* (pp. 413–427). New York: Plenum Press.

Gorelick, D. A., & Paredes, A. (1992). Effect of fluoxetine on alcohol consumption in male alcoholics. *Alcoholism: Clinical & Experimental Research, 16*, 261–265.

Gottheil, E., Thornton, C., & Weinstein, S. (2002). Effectiveness of high versus low structure individual counseling for substance abuse. *The American Journal on Addictions, 11*, 4, 279–290.

Graham, R., Wodak, A. D., & Whelan, G. (2002). New pharmacotherapies for alcohol dependence. *Medical Journal of Australia*, 177, 103–107.

Grant, B. F., & Harford, T. C. (1995). Comorbidity between DSM-IV alcohol use disorders and major depression: Results of a national survey. *Drug and Alcohol Dependence, 39*, 197–206.

Green, A. I., Noordsy, D. L., Brunette, M. F., & O'Keefe, C. (2008). Substance abuse and schizophrenia: Pharmacotherapeutic intervention. *Journal on Substance Abuse Treatment, 34*, 1, 61–71.

Griffith, J. D., Jasinski, D. R., Casten, G. P., & McKinney, G. R. (1986). Investigation of the abuse liability of buspirone in alcohol-dependent patients. *American Journal of Medicine, 80*(Suppl 3B), 30–35.

Guardia, J., Caso, C., Arias, F., Gual, A., Sanahuja, J., Ramirez, M., et al. (2002). A double-blind, placebo-controlled study of naltrexone in the treatment of alcohol-dependence disorder: Results from a multicenter clinical trial. *Alcohol: Clinical & Experimental Research, 26*, 1381–1387.

Haber, P. S. (2003). Liver disease. In A. W. Graham, T. K. Schultz, M. F. Mayo-Smith, R. K. Ries, & B. B. Wilford. (Eds.). *Principles of addiction medicine.* (3rd ed.). Chevy Chase, MD: American Society of Addiction Medicine.

Hague, W. H., Wilson, L. G., Dudley, D. L., & Cannon, D. S. (1976). Post-detoxification drug treatment of anxiety and depression in alcoholic addicts. *Journal of Nervous and Mental Diseases, 162*, 354–359.

Harwood, H. J. (2000). *Updating estimates of the economic costs of alcohol abuse in the United States: Estimates, update methods, and data.* Bethesda, MD: National Institute on Alcohol Abuse and Alcoholism.

Heinala, P., Alho, H., Kiianmaa, K., Lonngvist, J., Kuoppasalmi, K., & Sinclair, D. (2001). Targeted use of naltrexone without prior detoxification in the treatment of alcohol dependence: A factorial double-blind, placebo-controlled trial. *Journal of Clinical Psychopharmacology*, 21, 287–292.

Heinz, A., Siessmeier, T., Wrase, J., Hermann, D., Klein, S., Grusser, S. M., et al. (2004). Correlation between dopamine D2 receptors in the ventral striatum and central processing of alcohol cues and craving. *American Journal of Psychiatry, 161*, 1783–1789.

Hesselbrock, M. N., Meyer, R. E., & Keener, J. J. (1985). Psychopathology in hospitalized alcoholics. *Archives of General Psychiatry, 2*, 1050–1055.

Hillemacher, T., & Bleich, S. (2008). Neurobiology and treatment in alcoholism--Recent findings regarding Lesch's typology of alcohol dependence. *Alcohol and Alcoholism, 43*, 3, 341–346.

Ho, M. P., Yo, C. H., Liu C. M., Chen, C. L., & Lee, C. C. (2007). Refractive hypotension in a patient with disulfiram-ethanol reaction. *American Journal of the Medical Sciences, 333*, 1, 53–55.

Hoyumpa, A. M., & Schenker, S. (1982). Major drug interactions: Effect of liver disease, alcohol and malnutrition. *Annual Review of Medicine, 33*, 113–149.

Jacobson, A. F., Dominguez, R. A., Goldstein, B. J., & Steinbook, R. M. (1985). Comparison of buspirone and diazepam in generalized anxiety disorder. *Pharmacotherapy, 5*, 290–296.

Jaffe, J. H., Ciraulo, D. A., Nies, A., Dixon, R. B., & Monroe, L. L. (1983). Abuse potential of halazepam and diazepam in patients recently treated for acute alcohol withdrawal. *Clinical Pharmacology & Therapeutics, 34*, 623–630.

Jaffe, A. J., Rounsaville, B., Chang, G., Schottenfeld, R, S., Meyer, R. E., & O'Malley, S. S. (1996). Naltrexone, relapse prevention, and supportive therapy with alcoholics: an analysis of patient treatment matching. *Journal of Consulting and Clinical Psychology, 64*, 5, 1044–1053.

Jang, G. R., & Harris, R. Z. (2007). Drug interactions involving ethanol and alcoholic beverages. *Expert Opinion on Drug Metabolism and Toxicology, 3*, 5, 719–731.

Johnson, B. A. (2004). Uses of topiramate in the treatment of alcohol dependence. *Expert Reviews in Neurotherapy, 4*, 5, 751–758.

Johnson, B. A. (2005). Recent advances in the development of treatments for alcohol and cocaine dependence: Focus on topiramate and other modulators of GABA or glutamate function. *CNS Drugs, 19*, 10, 873–896.

Johnson, B. A. (2006). A synopsis of the pharmacological rationale, properties and therapeutic effects of depot preparations of naltrexone for treating alcohol dependence. *Expert Opinion in Pharmacotherapy, 7*, 8, 1065–1073.

Johnson, B. A. (2007). Naltrexone long-acting formulation in the treatment of alcohol dependence. *Therapeutics and Clinical Risk Management, 3*, 5, 741–749.

Johnson, B. A. (2008). Update on neuropharmacological treatments for alcoholism: Scientific basis and clinical findings. *Biochemical Pharmacology, 75*, 1, 34–56.

Johnson, B. A., Ait-Daoud, N., Bowden, C. L., DiClemente, C. C., Roache, J. D., Lawson, K., et al. (2003). Oral topiramate for treatment of alcohol dependence: a randomised controlled trial. *Lancet, 361*, 1677–1685.

Johnson, B. A., Roache, J. D., Javors, M. A., DiClemente, C. C., Cloninger, C. R., Prihoda, T. J., et al. (2000). Ondansetron for reduction of drinking among biologically predisposed alcoholic patients: A randomized controlled trial. *Journal of the American Medical Association*, 284, 963–971.

Johnson, B. A., Rosenthal, N., Capece, J. A., Wiegand, F., Mao, L., Beyers, K., et al (2007). Topiramate for treating alcohol dependence: A randomized controlled trial. *Journal of the American Medical Association, 298*, 14, 1641–1651.

Kabel, D. I., & Petty, F. (1996). A double blind study of fluoxetine in severe alcohol dependence: Adjunctive therapy during and after inpatient treatment. *Alcoholism: Clinical & Experimental Research*, 20, 780–784.

Kelly, J. F., & McCrady, B. S. (2008). Twelve-step facilitation in non-specialty settings. *Recent Developments in Alcoholism, 18*, 321–346.

Kenna, G. A. (2005). Pharmacotherapy of alcohol dependence: Targeting a complex disorder. *Drug Discovery Today: Therapeutic Strategies, 2*, 1, 71–78.

Kenna, G. A., McGeary, J. E., & Swift, R. M. (2004). Pharmacotherapy, pharmacogenomics, and the future of alcohol dependence treatment, part 1. *American Journal of Health-System Pharmacy, 61*, 21, 2272–2279.

Kessler, R. C., Crum, R. M., Warner, L. A., Nelson, C. B., Schulenberg, J., & Anthony, J. C. (1997). Lifetime co-occurrence of DSM-IIIR alcohol abuse and dependence with other psychiatric disorders in the National Comorbidity Study. *Archives of General Psychiatry, 54*, 313–321.

Kessler, R. C., McGonagle, K. A., Zhao, S., Nelson, C. B., Hughes, M., Eshleman, S., et al. (1994). Lifetime and 12-month prevalence of DSM-IIIR psychiatric disorders in the United States. *Archives of General Psychiatry, 51*, 8–19.

Kiefer, F., Jiménez-Arriero, M. A., Klein, O., Diehl, A., & Rubio, G. (2008). Cloninger's typology and treatment outcome in alcohol-dependent subjects during pharmacotherapy with naltrexone. *Addiction Biology, 13*, 1, 124–129.

Kiefer, F., & Mann, K. (2005). New achievements and pharmacotherapeutic approaches in the treatment of alcohol dependence. *European Journal of Pharmacology, 526*, 1–3, 163–71.

Kissin, B. (1977). Medical management of the alcoholic patient. In B. Kissin, & H. Begleiter. (Eds.). *The biology of alcoholism, Vol. 5. Treatment and rehabilitation of the chronic alcoholic.* (pp. 55–103). New York: Plenum Press.

Koch, M., & Banys, P. (2001). Liver transplantation and opioid dependence. *Journal of the American Medical Association, 285*, 8, 1056–1058.

Koob, G. F., Roberts, A. J., Schulteis, G., Parsons, L. H., Heyser, C. J., Hyytia, P., et al. (1998). Neurocircuitry targets in ethanol reward and dependence. *Alcoholism, Clinical and Experimental Research, 22*, 3–9.

Kranzler, H. R. (1995). *The pharmacology of alcohol abuse.* New York: Springer Publishing.

Kranzler, H. R. (2000). Pharmacotherapy of alcoholism: Gaps in knowledge and opportunities for research. *Alcohol and Alcoholism, 35*, 537–547.

Kranzler, H. R., Armeli, S., Tennen, H., Blomgvist, O., Oncken, C., Petry, N., et al. (2003). Targeted naltrexone for early problem drinkers. *Journal of Clinical Psychopharmacology, 23*, 3, 294–304.

Kranzler, H. R., Burleson, J. A., Korner, P., Del Boca, F. K., Bohn, M. J., Brown, J., et al. (1995). Placebo-controlled trial of fluoxetine as an adjunct to relapse prevention in alcoholics. *American Journal of Psychiatry, 152*, 391–397.

Kranzler, H. R., Burleson, J. A., Brown, J., & Babor, T. F. (1996). Fluoxetine treatment seems to reduce the beneficial effects of cognitive-behavioral therapy in Type B alcoholics. *Alcoholism: Clinical & Experimental Research, 20*, 1534–1541.

Kranzler, H. R., Del Boca, F., Korner, P., & Brown, J. (1993). Adverse effects limit the usefulness of fluvoxamine for the treatment of alcoholism. *Journal of Substance Abuse Treatment, 10*, 283–287.

Kranzler, H. R., & Jaffe, J. H. (2003). Pharmacologic interventions for alcoholism. In: A. W. Graham, T. K. Schultz, M. F. Mayo-Smith, R. K. Ries, & B. B. Wilford. (Eds.). *Principles of addiction medicine.* (3rd ed.). Chevy Chase, MD: American Society of Addiction Medicine.

Kranzler, H. R., Mason, B. J., Pettinati, H. M., & Anton, R. F. (1997). Methodological issues in pharmacotherapy trials with alcoholics. In: M. Hertzman, & D. Feltner. (Eds.). *The handbook of psychopharmacology trials.* (pp. 213–245). New York: New York University Press.

Kranzler, H. R., Modesto-Lowe, V., & Nuwayser, E. S. (1998). A sustained-release naltrexone preparation for treatment of alcohol dependence. *Alcoholism: Clinical & Experimental Research, 22*, 1074–1079.

Kranzler, H. R., & Rounsaville, B. J. (Eds.) (1998). *Dual diagnosis: Substance abuse and comorbid medical and psychiatric disorders.* New York: Marcel Dekker.

Kranzler, H. R., Stephenson, J. J., Montejano, L., Wang, S., & Gastfriend, D. R. (2008). Persistence with oral naltrexone for alcohol treatment: Implications for health-care utilization. *Addiction, 103*, 11, 1801–1808.

Kranzler, H. R., Tennen, H., Penta, C., & Bohn, M. J. (1997). Targeted naltrexone treatment in early problem drinkers. *Addictive Behaviors, 22*, 431–436.

Kranzler, H. R., & Van Kirk, J. (2001). Efficacy of naltrexone and acamprosate for alcoholism treatment: A meta-analysis. *Alcohol: Clinical & Experimental Research, 25*, 1335–1341.

Kranzler, H. R., Wesson, D. R., Billot, L., DrugAbuse Sciences Naltrexone Depot Study Group. (2004). Naltrexone depot for treatment of alcohol dependence: A multicenter, randomized, placebo-controlled clinical trial. *Alcohol: Clinical & Experimental Research, 28*, 7, 1051–1059.

Krystal, J. H., Cramer, J. A., Krol, W. F., Kirk, G. F., Rosenheck, R. A., Veterans Affairs Naltrexone Cooperative Study et al. (2001). Naltrexone in the treatment of alcohol dependence. *New England Journal of Medicine, 345*, 1734–1739.

Laaksonen, E., Koski-Jännes, A., Salaspuro, M., Ahtinen, H., & Alho, H. (2008). A randomized, multicentre, open-label, comparative trial of disulfiram, naltrexone and acamprosate in the treatment of alcohol dependence. *Alcohol and Alcoholism, 43*, 1, 53–61.

LeMarquand, D., Pihl, R. O., & Benkelfat, C. (1994a). Serotonin and alcohol intake, abuse, and dependence: Findings of animal studies. *Biological Psychiatry, 36*, 395–421.

LeMarquand, D., Pihl, R. O., & Benkelfat, C. (1994b). Serotonin and alcohol intake, abuse, and dependence: Clinical evidence. *Biological Psychiatry, 36*, 326–337.

Lhuintre, J. P., Daoust, M., Moore, N. D., Chretien, P., Saligaut, C., Tran, G., et al. (1985). Ability of calcium bis acetyl homotaurinate, a GABA agonist, to prevent relapse in weaned alcoholics. *Lancet, 1*, 1014–1016.

Lhuintre, J. P., Moore, N., Tran, G., Steru, L., Langrenon, S., Daoust, M., et al. (1990). Acamprosate appears to decrease alcohol intake in weaned alcoholics. *Alcohol & Alcoholism, 25*, 613–622.

Li, T. K. (2000). Clinical perspectives for the study of craving and relapse in animal models. *Addiction, 95*, Suppl. 2, S55–S60.

Lindros, K. O., Stowell, A., Pikkarainen, P., & Salaspuro, M. (1981). The disulfiram (Antabuse)-Alcohol reaction in male alcoholics: its efficient management by 4-methylpyrazole. *Alcoholism, Clinical and Experimental Research, 5*, 4, 528–530.

Litten, R. Z., Fertig, J., Mattson M., & Egli, M. (2005). Development of medications for alcohol use disorders: Recent advances and ongoing challenges. *Expert Opinions on Emerging Drugs*, 10, 2, 323–343.

Lucey, M. R., Silverman, B. L., Illeperuma, A., & O'Brien, C. P. (2008). Hepatic safety of once-monthly injectable extended-release naltrexone administered to actively drinking alcoholics. *Alcoholism, Clinical and Experimental Research, 32*, 3, 498–504.

Maisto, S. A., Clifford, P. R., Stout, R. L., & Davis, C. M. (2008). Factors mediating the association between drinking in the first year after alcohol treatment and drinking at three years. *Journal of Studies on Alcohol and Drugs, 69*, 5, 728–737.

Major, L. F., Lerner, P., Ballenger, J. K., Brown, G. L., Goodwin, F. K., & Lovenberg, W. (1979). Dopamine beta-hydroxylase in the cerebrospinal fluid: Relationship to disulfiram induced psychosis. *Biological Psychiatry, 14*, 337–344.

Malcolm, R., Olive, M. F., & Lechner, W. (2008). The safety of disulfiram for the treatment of alcohol and cocaine dependence in randomized clinical trials: Guidance for clinical practice. *Expert Opinion on Drug Safety, 7*, 4, 459–472.

Mann, K. (2004). Pharmacotherapy of alcohol dependence: A review of the clinical data. *CNS Drugs*, 18, 8, 485–504.

Mann, K., Kiefer, F., Spanagel, R., & Littleton, J. (2008). Acamprosate: Recent findings and future research directions. *Alcoholism, Clinical and Experimental Research, 32*, 7, 1105–1110.

Mannelli, P., Peindl, K., Masand, P. S., & Patkar, A. A. (2007). Long-acting injectable naltrexone for the treatment of alcohol dependence. *Expert Review of Neurotherapies, 7*, 10, 1265–1277.

Mansell, D., Penk, W., Hankin, C. S., Lee, A., Spiro, A., Skinner, K. M, et al. (2006). The illness burden of alcohol-related disorders among VA patients: The veterans health study. *Journal of Ambulatory Care Management, 29*, 1, 61–70.

Marlatt, G. A. (1996a). Taxonomy of high-risk situations for alcohol relapse: evolution and development of a cognitive-behavioral model. *Addiction, 91*, Suppl. 1, S37–S49.

Marlatt, G. A. (1996b). Lest taxonomy become taxidermy: a comment on the relapse replication and extension project. *Addiction, 91*, Suppl. 1, 147–154.

Marlatt, G. A., Barrett, K., & Daley, D. C. (1999). Relapse prevention. In: M. Galanter, & H. D. Kleber. (eds.) *Textbook of substance abuse.* (2nd ed., pp. 353–365). Washington, DC: American Psychiatric Press.

Marlatt, G. A., & Gordon, J. R. (1985). *Relapse prevention: maintenance strategies in the treatment of addictive behaviors.* New York: Guilford Press.

Mason, B. J. (2006). Acamprosate for alcohol dependence: An update for the clinician. *Focus, 4*, 505–511.

Mason, B. J. (2005a). Acamprosate in the treatment of alcohol dependence. *Expert Opinions on Pharmacotherapy, 6*, 12, 2103–2115.

Mason, B. J. (2005b). Rationale for combining acamprosate and naltrexone for treating alcohol dependence. *Journal of Studies on Alcohol, 15*, 148–156.

Mason, B. J. (2001). Treatment of alcohol-dependent outpatients with acamprosate: A clinical review. *Journal of Clinical Psychiatry, 62*, (Suppl 20), 42–48.

Mason, B., & Goodman, A. (2000). Acamprosate: New preclinical and clinical research. Presented at the 23rd Annual Scientific Meeting of the Research Society on Alcoholism, Denver, Colorado, June 24.

Mason, B. J., & Ownby, R. L. (2000). Acamprosate for the treatment of alcohol dependence: a review of double-blind, placebo-controlled trials. *CNS Spectrums, 5*, 2, 58–69.

Mason, B. J., Ritvo, E. C., Morgan, R. O., Salvato, F. R., Goldberg, G., Welch B, et al. (1994). A double-blind, placebo-controlled pilot study to evaluate the efficacy and safety of oral nalmefene HCL for alcohol dependence. *Alcoholism: Clinical & Experimental Research, 18*, 1162–1167.

Mason, B. J., Salvato, F. R., Williams, L. D., Ritvo, C. E., & Cutler, R. B. (1999). A double-blind, placebo-controlled study of oral nalmefene for alcohol dependence. *Archives of General Psychiatry, 56*, 719–724.

Mattila, M. J., Aranko, K., & Seppala, T. (1982). Acute effects of buspirone and alcohol on psychomotor skills. *Journal of Clinical Psychiatry, 43*, 56–60.

Mattson, M. E., & Litten, R. Z. (2005). Combining treatments for alcoholism: Why and how? *Journal of Studies on Alcohol, 15*, 8–16.

McCaul, M. E., Wand, G. S., Rohde, C., & Lee, S. M. (2000). Serum 6-beta-naltrexol levels are related to alcohol responses in heavy drinkers. *Alcoholism: Clinical & Experimental Research*, 24, 1385–1391.

Meza, E., & Kranzler, H. R. (1996). Closing the gap between alcoholism research and practice: The case for pharmacotherapy. *Psychiatric Services, 47*, 917–920.

Milne, H. J., & Parke, T. R. (2007). Hypotension and ST depression as a result of disulfiram ethanol reaction. *European Journal of Emergency Medicine, 14*, 4, 228–229.

Morley, K. C., Teesson, M., Reid, S. C., Sannibale, C., Thomson, C., Phung, N., et al. (2006). Naltrexone versus acamprosate in the treatment of alcohol dependence: A multi-centre, randomized, double-blind, placebo-controlled trial. *Addiction, 101*, 10, 1451–1462.

Mullaney, J. A., & Trippett, C. J. (1979). Alcohol dependence and phobias: Clinical description and relevance. *Psychiatry, 135*, 565–573.

Myers, R. D., Borg, S., & Mossberg, R. (1986). Antagonism by naltrexone of voluntary alcohol selection in the chronically drinking macaque monkey. *Alcoholism, 3*, 6, 383–388.

Myrick, H., & Anton, R. F. (2004). Recent advances in the pharmacotherapy of alcoholism. *Current Psychiatry Reports, 6*, 5, 332–338.

Myrick, H., Anton, R. F., Li, X., Henderson, S., Randall, P. K., & Voronin, K. (2008). Effect of naltrexone and ondansetron on alcohol cue-induced activation of the ventral striatum in alcohol-dependent people. *Archives of General Psychiatry, 65*, 4, 466–475.

Myrick, H., Brady, K. T., & Malcolm, R. (2001). New developments in the pharmacotherapy of alcohol dependence. *American Journal on Addictions, 10*, (Suppl), 3–15.

Myrick, H., Anton, R. F., Li, X., Henderson, S., Drobes, D., Voronin, K., et al. (2004). Differential brain activity in alcoholics and social drinkers to alcohol cues: Relationship to craving. *Neuropsychopharmacology, 29*, 393–402.

Nace, C. P., Saxon, J. J., & Shore, N. (1983). A comparison of borderline and nonborderline alcoholic patients. *Archives of General Psychiatry, 40*, 54–56.

Naranjo, C. A., Bremner, K. E. & Lanctot, K. L. (1995). Effects of citalopram and a brief psycho-social intervention on alcohol intake, dependence, and problems. *Addiction, 90*, 87–99.

Naranjo, C. A., Kadlec, K. E., Sanhueza, P., Woodley-Remus, D., & Sellers, E. M. (1990). Fluoxetine differentially alters alcohol intake and other consummatory behaviors in problem drinkers. *Clinical Pharmacology and Therapeutics, 47*, 490–498.

Naranjo, C. A., Poulos, C. X., Bremner, K. E., & Lanctot, K. L. (1992). Citalopram decreases desirability, liking, and consumption of alcohol in alcohol-dependent drinkers. *Clinical Pharmacology and Therapeutics, 51*, 729–739.

Naranjo, C. A., Sellers, E. M., Roach, C. A., Woodley, D. V., Sanchez-Craig, M., & Sykora, K. (1984). Zimelidine-induced variations in alcohol intake by nondepressed heavy drinkers. *Clinical Pharmacology and Therapeutics, 35*, 374–381.

Naranjo, C. A., Sellers, E. M., Sullivan, J. T., Woodley, D. V., Kadlec, K., & Sykora, K. (1987). The serotonin uptake inhibitor citalopram attenuates ethanol intake. *Clinical Pharmacology and Therapeutics, 41*, 266–274.

Naranjo, C. A., Sullivan, J. T., Kadlec, K. E., Woodley-Remus, D. V., Kennedy, G., & Sellers, E. M. (1989). Differential effects of viqualine on alcohol intake and other consummatory behaviors. *Clinical Pharmacology and Therapeutics, 46*, 301–309.

National Institute on Alcohol Abuse and Alcoholism. (2008). Helping patients who drink too much: A clinician's guide. Bethesda, MD: NIAAA, National Institutes of Health. Available online at: http://www.niaaa.nih.gov/Publications/EducationTrainingMaterials/guide.htm. Accessed September 17, 2009.

Neto, D., Lambaz, R., Aguiar, P., & Chick, J. (2008). Effectiveness of sequential combined treatment in comparison with treatment as usual in preventing relapse in alcohol dependence. *Alcohol and Alcoholism, 43*, 6, 661–668.

Nunes, E. V., & Levin, F. R. (2004). Treatment of depression in patients with alcohol and other drug dependence: a meta-analysis. *Journal of the American Medical Association, 291*, 1887–1896.

O'Brien, C. P. (2005). Anticraving medications for relapse prevention: A possible new class of psychoactive medications. *American Journal of Psychiatry*, 162, 8, 1423–1431.

O'Brien, C. P. (2006). Pharmacotherapies in the treatment of alcohol dependence (CME program). Annual Medical-Scientific Conference of the American Society of Addiction Medicine. San Diego, CA, May 6.

O'Malley, S. S., Garbutt, J. C., Gastfriend, D. R., Dong, Q., & Kranzler, H. R. (2007). Efficacy of extended-release naltrexone in alcohol-dependent patients who are abstinent before treatment. *Journal of Clinical Psychopharmacology, 27*, 5, 507–512.

O'Malley, S. S., Jaffe, A. J., Chang, G., Schottenfeld, R. S., Meyer, R. E., & Rounsaville, B. (1992). Naltrexone and coping skills therapy for alcohol dependence: A controlled study. *Archives of General Psychiatry, 49*, 894–898.

O'Malley, S. S., Jaffe, A. J., Chang, G., Rode, S., Schottenfeld, R., Meyer, R. E., et al. (1996). Six-month follow-up of naltrexone and psychotherapy for alcohol dependence. *Archives of General Psychiatry, 53*, 217–224.

O'Malley, S. S., Jaffe, A. J., Rode, S., & Rounsaville, B. J. (1996). Experience of a "slip" among alcoholics treated with naltrexone or placebo. *American Journal of Psychiatry, 153*, 281–283.

O'Malley, S. S., Krishnan-Sarin, S., Farren, C., Sinha, R., & Kreek, M. J. (2002). Naltrexone decreases craving and alcohol self-administration in alcohol-dependent subjects and activates the hypothalamo-pituitary-adreno-cortical axis. *Psychopharmacology (Berl.), 164*, 2, 239–240.

O'Malley, S. S., Rounsaville, B. J., Farren, C., Namkoong, K., Wu, R., Robinson, J., & O'Connor, P. G. (2003). Initial and maintenance naltrexone treatment for alcohol dependence using primary care vs specialty care: A nested sequence of 3 randomized trials. *Archives of Internal Medicine, 163*, 14, 1695–1704.

Oslin, D. W., Berrettini, W., Kranzler, H. R., Pettinati, H., Gelernter, J., Volpicelli, J. R., et al. (2003). A functional polymorphism of the mu-opioid receptor gene is associated with therapeutic response in alcohol dependent patients treated with naltrexone. *Neuropsychopharmacology, 28*, 1546–1552.

Oslin, D. W., Lynch, K. G., Pettinati, H. M., Kampman, K. M., Gariti, P., Gelfand, L., et al. (2008). A placebo-controlled randomized clinical trial of naltrexone in the context of different levels of psychosocial intervention. *Alcohol Clin Exp Research, 32*, 7, 1299–1308.

Pagano, M. E., Zemore, S. E., Onder, C. C., & Stout, R. L. (2009). Predictors of initial AA-related helping: Findings from Project MATCH. *Journal of Studies on Alcohol and Drugs, 70*, 1, 117–125.

Paille, F. M., Guelfi, J. D., Perkins, A. C., Royer, R. J., Steru, L., & Parot, P. (1995). Double-blind randomized multicentre trial of acamprosate in maintaining abstinence from alcohol. *Alcohol & Alcoholism, 30*, 239–247.

Passeri, L. A., Ellis, E., & Sinn, D. P. (1993). Relationship of substance abuse to complications with mandibular fractures. *Journal of Oral and Maxillofacial Surgeons, 51*, 22–25.

Peachey, J. E., Brien, J. F., Zilm, D. H., Loomis, C. W., Hemy, M. F., & Maglana, S. M. (1981). The calcium cyanamide-ethanol interaction in man. Effects of repeated ethanol administration. *Journal of Studies on Alcohol, 42*, 3, 208–216.

Peachey, J. E., Maglana, S., Robinson, G. M., Hemy, M. & Brien, J. F. (1981). Cardiovascular changes during the calcium carbimide-ethanol interaction. *Clinical Pharmacology and Therapeutics, 29*, 1, 40–46.

Pelc, I., Le Bon, O., Lebert, P., et al. (1996). Acamprosate in the treatment of alcohol dependence: A 6-month post-detoxification study. In M. Soyka. (Ed.). *Acamprosate in relapse prevention of alcoholism.* (pp. 133–142). Berlin: Springer-Verlag.

Pelc, I., Verbanck, P., Le Bon, O., Gavrilovic, M., Lion, K., & Lehert, P. (1997). Efficacy and safety of acamprosate in the treatment of detoxified alcohol-dependent patients. A 90-day placebo-controlled dose-finding study. *British Journal of Psychiatry, 171*, 73–77.

Penberthy, J. K., Ait-Daoud, N., Breton, M., Kovatchev, B., DiClemente, C. C., & Johnson, B. A. (2007). Evaluating readiness and treatment seeking effects in a pharmacotherapy trial for alcohol dependence. *Alcohol, Clinical and Experimental Research, 31*, 9, 1538–1544.

Peterson, A. M. (2007). Improving adherence in patients with alcohol dependence: A new role for pharmacists. *American Journal of Health-System Pharmacy, 64*, (5 Suppl 3), S23–29.

Petrakis, I. L., Nich, C., & Ralevski, E. (2006). Psychotic spectrum disorders and alcohol abuse: a review of pharmacotherapeutic strategies and a report on the effectiveness of naltrexone and disulfiram. *Schizophrenia Bulletin, 32*, 4, 644–654.

Petrakis, I. L., O'Malley, S., & Rounsaville, B. (2004) Naltrexone augmentation of neuroleptic treatment in alcohol abusing patients with schizophrenia. *Psychopharmacology, 172*, 291–297.

Petrakis, I. L., Poling, J., Levinson, C., Nich, C., Carroll, K., Ralevski, E., et al. (2006). Naltrexone and disulfiram in patients with alcohol dependence and comorbid post-traumatic stress disorder. *Biological Psychiatry, 60*, 7, 777–783.

Petrakis, I., Ralevski, E., Nich, C., Levinson, C., Carroll, K., Poling, J., et al. (2007). Naltrexone and disulfiram in patients with alcohol dependence and current depression. *Journal of Clinical Psychopharmacology, 27*, 2, 160–165.

Pettinati, H. M., Gastfriend, D. R., Dong, Q., Kranzler, H. R., O'Malley, S. S. (2009). Effect of extended-release naltrexone (XR-NTX) on quality of life in alcohol-dependent patients. *Alcoholism, Clinical and Experimental Research, 33*, 350–356.

Pettinati, H. M., Kampman, K. M., Lynch, K. G., Xie, H., Dackis, C., Rabinowitz, A. R., et al. (2008). A double blind, placebo-controlled trial that combines disulfiram and naltrexone for treating co-occurring cocaine and alcohol dependence. *Addictive Behaviors, 33*, 5, 651–667.

Pettinatti, H. M., Kampman, K. M., Macfadden, W., et al. (2006). Randomized, placebo controlled trial of quetiapine for the treatment of alcohol dependence. (Abstract No 47). *Alcohol Clin Exp Res, 30*, 108A.

Pettinati, H. M., & Rabinowitz, A. R. (2005). Recent advances in the treatment of alcoholism. *Clinical Neuroscience Research, 5*, 151–159.

Pettinati, H. M., Volpicelli, J. R., Kranzler, H. R., Luck, G., Rukstalis, M. R., & Cnaan, A. (2000). Sertraline treatment for alcohol dependence: Interactive effects of medication and subtype. *Alcoholism: Clinical & Experimental Research, 24*, 1041–1049.

Pettinati, H. M., Volpicelli, J. R., Pierce, J. D. Jr., & O'Brien, C. P. (2000). Improving naltrexone response: An intervention for medical practitioners to enhance medication compliance in alcohol dependent patients. *Journal of Addictive Diseases, 19*, 71–83.

Poldrugo, F. (1997). Acamprosate treatment in a long-term community-based alcohol rehabilitation programme. *Addiction, 92*, 1537–1546.

Project MATCH Research Group. (1997). Matching alcoholism treatments to client heterogeneity: Project MATCH posttreatment drinking outcomes. *Journal of Studies on Alcohol, 58*, 7–29.

Regier, D. A., Farmer, M. E., Rae, D. S., Locke, B. Z., Keith, S. J., Judd, L. L., et al. (1990). Comorbidity of mental disorders with alcohol and other drug abuse. Results from the Epidemiologic Catchment Area (ECA) Study. *Journal of the American Medical Association, 264*, 2511–2518.

Richardson, K., Baillie, A., Reid, S., Morley, K., Teesson, M., Sannibale, C., et al. (2008). Do acamprosate or naltrexone have an effect on daily drinking by reducing craving for alcohol? *Addiction, 103*, 6, 953–959.

Rimondini, R., Arlinde, C., Sommer, W., & Heilig, M. (2002). Long-lasting increase in voluntary ethanol consumption and transcriptional regulation in the rat brain after intermittent exposure to alcohol. *The FASEB Journal, 16*, 1, 27–35.

Roberts, J. S., Anton, R. F., Latham, P. K., & Moak, D. H. (1999). Factor structure and predictive validity of the Obsessive Compulsive Drinking Scale. *Alcoholism: Clinical and Experimental Research, 23*, 1484–1491.

Roozen, H. G., de Waart, R., & van den Brink, W. (2007). Efficacy and tolerability of naltrexone in the treatment of alcohol dependence: Oral versus injectable delivery. *European Addiction Research, 13*, 4, 201–206.

Rosenthal, R. N. (2006). Pharmacotherapies in the treatment of alcohol dependence (CME program). Annual Medical-Scientific Conference of the American Society of Addiction Medicine, San Diego, California, May 6.

Rösner, S., Leucht, S., Lehert, P., & Soyka, M. (2008). Acamprosate supports abstinence, naltrexone prevents excessive drinking: Evidence from a meta-analysis with unreported outcomes. *Journal of Psychopharmacology, 22*, 1, 11–23.

Ross, H. E., Glaser, F. B., & Germanson, T. (1988). The prevalence of psychiatric disorders in patients with alcohol and other drug problems. *Archives of General Psychiatry, 45*, 1023–1031.

Roussaux, J. P., Hers, D., & Ferauge, M. (1996). Does acamprosate diminish the appetite for alcohol in weaned alcoholics? [in French]. *Journal de Pharmacie de Belgique, 51*, 65–68.

Samet, J. H., Walley, A. Y., & Bridden, C. (2007). Illicit drugs, alcohol, and addiction in human immunodeficiency virus. *Panminerva Medica, 49*, 2, 67–77 (Review).

Sands, B. F., Knapp, C. M., & Ciraulo, D. A. (1995). Interaction of alcohol with therapeutic drugs and drugs of abuse. In H. R. Kranzler. (Ed.). *The pharmacology of alcohol abuse*. (pp. 475–512). New York: Springer-Verlag.

Sass, H., Soyka, M., Mann, K., & Zieglgansberger, W. (1996). Relapse prevention by acamprosate: Results from a placebo controlled study on alcohol dependence. *Archives of General Psychiatry, 53*, 673–680.

Schuckit, M. (1983). Alcoholic patients with secondary depression. *American Journal of Psychiatry, 140*, 711–714.

Schuckit, M. A. (2009). An overview of genetic influences in alcoholism. *Journal of Substance Abuse Treatmeant, 36*, 1, S5–14.

Scott, L. J., Figgitt, D. P., Keam, S. J., & Waugh, J. (2005). Acamprosate: A review of its use in the maintenance of abstinence in patients with alcohol dependence. *CNS Drugs, 19*, 5, 445–464.

Sellers, E. M., Naranjo, C. A., & Peachey, J. E. (1981). Drugs to decrease alcohol consumption. *New England Journal of Medicine, 305*, 1255–1262.

Seppala, T., Aranko, K., Mattila, M. J., & Shrotriya, R. C. (1982). Effects of alcohol on buspirone and lorazepam actions. *Clinical Pharmacology and Therapeutics, 32*, 201–207.

Shea, C. W. (2008). From the neurobiologic basis of alcohol dependency to pharmacologic treatment strategies: Bridging the knowledge gap. *The Southern Medical Journal, 101*, 2, 179–185.

Snyder, J. L., & Bowers, T. G. (2008). The efficacy of acamprosate and naltrexone in the treatment of alcohol dependence: A relative benefits analysis of randomized controlled trials. *American Journal of Drug and Alcohol Abuse, 34*, 4, 449–461.

Sokolow, L., Welte, J., Hynes, G., & Lyons, J. (1981). Multiple substance use by alcoholics. *British Journal of Addiction, 76*, 147–158.

Soyka, M., Kranzler, H. R., Berglund, M., Gorelick, D., Hesselbrock, V., Johnson, B. A., et al. (2008). World Federation of Societies of Biological Psychiatry (WFSBP) Guidelines for Biological Treatment of Substance Use and Related Disorders, Part 1: Alcoholism. *The World Journal of Biological Psychiatry, 9*, 1, 6–23.

Spanagel, R., & Kiefer, F. (2008). Drugs for relapse prevention of alcoholism: Ten years of progress. *Trends in Pharmacological Sciences*, 29, 3, 109–115.

Spies, C., Tonnesen, H., Andreasson, S., Helander, A., & Conigrave, K. (2001). Perioperative morbidity and mortality in chronic alcoholic patients. *Alcoholism: Clinical & Experimental Research, 25*, 5, 164S–170S.

Srisurapanont, M., & Jarusuraisin, N. (2005a). Naltrexone for the treatment of alcoholism: A meta-analysis of randomized controlled trials. *International Journal of Neuropsychopharmacology, 8*, 2, 267–280.

Srisurapanont, M., & Jarusuraisin, N. (2005b). Cochrane review: Opioid antagonists for alcohol dependence. *The Cochrane Database of Systematic Reviews, 1*, CD001867.

Starzl, T. E., Van, T. D., Tzakis, A. G., Iwatsuki, S., Todo, S., Marsh, J. W., et al. (1988). Orthotopic liver transplantation for alcoholic cirrhosis. *Journal of the American Medical Association, 260*, 17, 2542–2544.

Stitzer, M., & Petry, N. (2006). Contingency management for treatment of substance abuse. *Annual Review of Clinical Psychology, 2*, 411–434.

Stowe, J., & Kotz, M. (2001). Addiction medicine in organ transplantation. *Progress in Transplantation, 11*, 1, 50–57.

Streeton, C., & Whelan, G. (2001). Naltrexone, a relapse prevention maintenance treatment of alcohol dependence: A meta-analysis of randomized controlled trials. *Alcohol & Alcoholism, 36*, 544–552.

Swift, R. M. (1999). Drug therapy for alcohol dependence. *New England Journal of Medicine, 340*, 1482–490.

Swift, R. (2007). Emerging approaches to managing alcohol dependence. *American Journal of Health System Pharmacy*, 64, S12–2.

Swift, R., & Pettinati, H. M. (2005). Choosing pharmacotherapies for the COMBINE Study – Process and procedures: An investigational approach to combination pharmacotherapy for the treatment of alcohol dependence. *Journal of Studies on Alcohol*, 15, 141–47.

Tambour, S., & Quertemont, E. (2007). Preclinical and clinical pharmacology of alcohol dependence. *Fundamentals of Clinical Pharmacology, 21*, 1, 9–28.

Tempesta, E., Janiri, L., Bignamini, A., Chabac, S., & Potgieter, A. (2000). Acamprosate and relapse prevention in the treatment of alcohol dependence: A placebo-controlled study. *Alcohol and Alcoholism, 35*, 202–209.

Tiihonen, J., Ryynanen, O-P., Kauhanen, J., Hakola, H. P, & Salaspuro, M. (1996). Citalopram in the treatment of alcoholism: A double-blind placebo-controlled study. *Pharmacopsychiatry, 29*, 27–29.

Tollefson, G. D., Montague-Clouse, J., & Tollefson, S. L. (1992). Treatment of comorbid generalized anxiety in a recently detoxified alcohol population with a selective serotonergic drug (Buspirone). *Journal of Clinical Psychopharmacology, 12*, 19–26.

Tonnesen, H. (1992). Influence of alcohol on several physiological functions and its reversibility: A surgical view. *Acta Psychiatrica Scandinavica, 86*, 67–71.

Torrens, M., Fonseca, F., Mateu, G., & Farre, M. (2005). Efficacy of antidepressants in substance use disorders with and without comorbid depression: a systematic review and meta-analysis. *Drug and Alcohol Dependence, 78*, 1–22.

Tsui, J. I., Pletcher, M. J., Vittinghoff, E., Seal, K., & Gonzales, R. (2006). Hepatitis C and hospital outcomes in patients admitted with alcohol-related problems. *Journal of Hepatology, 44*, 2, 262–266.

Volkow, N. D., & Fowler, J. S. (2000). Addiction, a disease of compulsion and drive: involvement of the orbitofrontal cortex. *Cerebral Cortex, 10*, 318–325.

Volkow, N. D., & Li, T. K. (2005). Drugs and alcohol: Treating and preventing abuse, addiction and their medical consequences. *Pharmacologic Therapies, 108*, 1, 3–17.

Volpicelli, J., Alterman, A. I., Hayashida, A., & O'Brien, C. (1992). Naltrexone in the treatment of alcohol dependence. *Archives of General Psychiatry, 49*, 867–880.

Volpicelli, J. R., Pettinati, H. M., McLellan, A. T. et al. (2001). *Combining medication and psychosocial treatments for addiction—The Brenda Approach.* New York: Guilford.

Volpicelli, J., Rhines, K. C., Rhines, J. S., Volpicelli, L. A., Alterman, A. I., & O'Brien, C. P. (1997). Naltrexone and alcohol dependence: Role of subject compliance. *Archives of General Psychiatry, 54*, 737–742.

Volpicelli, J. R., Watson, N. T., King, A.C., Sherman, C. E., & O'Brien, C. P. (1995). Effect of naltrexone on alcohol "high" in alcoholics. *American Journal of Psychiatry, 152*, 613–615.

Weaver, M. F. (2003). Management of the addicted woman in pregnancy. In A. W. Graham, T. K. Schultz, M. F. Mayo-Smith, R. K. Ries, & B. B. Wilford. (Eds.). *Principles of addiction medicine.* (3rd ed.). Chevy Chase, MD: American Society of Addiction Medicine.

West, S. L., Garbutt, J. C., Carey, T. S. et al. (1999). *Pharmacotherapy for alcohol dependence.* Rockville, MD: Agency for Health Care Policy and Research.

Wikler, A. (1980). A theory of opioid dependence. *NIDA Research Monograph, 30*, 174–178.

Williams, S. H. (2005). Medications for treating alcohol dependence (review). *American Family Physician*, 72, 9, 1775–1780.

Wilson, A., Davidson, W. J., & Blanchard, R. (1980). Disulfiram implantation: A trial using placebo implants and two types of controls. *Journal of Studies on Alcohol, 41*, 429–436.

Wilson, S. T., Fertuck, E. A., Kwitel, A., Stanley, M. C., & Stanley, B. (2006). Impulsivity, suicidality and alcohol use disorders in adolescents and young adults with borderline personality disorder. *International Journal of Adolescent Medicine and Health, 18*, 1, 189–196.

Wolf, B., Iguchi, M. Y., & Griffiths, R. R. (1990). Sedative/tranquilizer use and abuse in alcoholics currently in outpatient treatment: Incidence, pattern and preference. In L. S. Harris. (Ed.). *Problems of drug dependence 1989.* (pp. 376–377). NIDA Research Monograph No. 95. Rockville, MD: National Institute on Drug Abuse.

Wood, D., Wender, P. H., & Reimherr, F. W. (1983). The prevalence of attention deficit disorder, residual type, or minimal brain dysfunction, in a population of male alcoholic patients. *American Journal of Psychiatry, 140*, 95–98.

Yourick, J. J., & Faiman, M. D. (1991). Disulfiram metabolism as a requirement for the inhibition of rat liver mitochondrial low Km aldehyde dehydrogenase. *Biochemical Pharmacology, 42*, 1361–1366.

Zweben, A., Pettinati, H. M., Weiss, R. D., Youngblood, M., Cox, C. E., Mattson, M. E., et al. (2008). Relationship between medication adherence and treatment outcomes: The COMBINE study. *Alcohol, Clinical and Experimental Research, 32*, 9, 1661–1669.

CHAPTER 6

Placement Criteria for Preventing and Managing Relapse

TREATMENT LEVELS WITHIN DIMENSION 5

The ASAM Patient Placement Criteria conceptualize treatment as a continuum marked by five basic levels of care, which are numbered in Roman numerals from Levels 0.5 through Level IV. Thus, the ASAM Criteria provide the addiction field with a nomenclature for describing the continuum of addiction services available to help the patient achieve an efficient, effective, and safe outcome.

Within each level of care, a decimal number (ranging from 0.1 to 0.9) expresses gradations of intensity within the existing levels of care. The ASAM Criteria thus describe gradations within each level of care. For example, a II.1 level of care (Intensive Outpatient Treatment) provides a benchmark for intensity at the minimum description of Level II care. This structure allows improved precision of description and better inter-rater reliability.

Level 0.5: Early Intervention

Early intervention is an organized service that may be delivered in a wide variety of settings. Early intervention services are designed to explore and address problems or risk factors that appear to be related to substance use and to help the individual recognize the harmful consequences of inappropriate substance use.

Length of Service

Length of service at Level 0.5 varies according to (a) an individual's ability to comprehend the information provided and use that information to make behavior changes and avoid problems related to substance use or (b) the appearance of new problems that require treatment at another level of care.

Level I: Outpatient Treatment

Level I encompasses organized outpatient treatment services, which may be delivered in a wide variety of settings. In Level I programs, addiction treatment staff, including addiction-credentialed physicians, provide professionally directed evaluation, treatment, and recovery services. Such services are provided in regularly scheduled sessions of (usually) fewer than 9 contact hours a week. The services follow a defined set of policies and procedures or clinical protocols.

Level I services are tailored to each patient's level of clinical severity and are designed to help the patient achieve changes in his or her alcohol- or other drug-using behaviors. Treatment thus must address major lifestyle, attitudinal, and behavioral issues that have the potential to undermine the goals of treatment or to impair the individual's ability to cope with major life tasks without the nonmedical use of alcohol or other drugs.

Level I services are appropriate in several different situations:

- Level I may be the initial level of care for a patient whose severity of illness warrants this intensity of treatment. Such a patient should be able to complete professionally directed addiction treatment at this level, thus using only one level of care, unless (a) an unanticipated event causes a change in his or her level of functioning, leading to a reassessment of the appropriateness of this level of care, or (b) there is recurring evidence of the patient's inability to use this level of care (such as repeated episodes of drinking or nonmedical drug use even after the treatment plan has been reviewed and revised).
- Level I may represent a "step down" from a more intensive level of care for a patient whose progress warrants such a transfer, assuming that he or she meets the criteria for placement in Level I.
- Level I may be used for a patient who is in the early stages of change and who is not yet ready to commit to full recovery (Dimension 4 issues). For such a patient, placement in a more intensive level of care is apt to lead to increased conflict, passive compliance, or even leaving treatment.

The relationship between the severity of illness and the intensity of treatment is most clearly seen in Dimensions 1, 2, and 3. On the other hand, increasing the intensity of services solely because of Dimension 4 issues may be counterproductive. An alternative approach is to use Level I services to engage the resistant individual in treatment. If this approach proves successful, the patient may no longer require a higher intensity of service, or may be able to better use such services.

Length of Service

The duration of treatment varies with the severity of the individual's illness and his or her response to treatment.

Co-Occurring Mental and Substance-Related Disorders

Level I services are appropriate for patients with co-occurring mental and substance-related disorders *if*:

1. The patient's disorders are of moderate severity (as defined in the introduction to this section) and have responded to more intensive treatment services. The mental disorders have resolved to an extent that addiction treatment services are assessed as potentially beneficial. However, ongoing monitoring of the patient's mental status is required.
2. The patient's disorders are of chronically *high severity* and are persistent, but are of low acuity and have stabilized to such an extent that integrated mental health and addiction treatment services are assessed as potentially beneficial. Patients who have severe and persistent mental

disorders may not have been able to achieve sobriety or to maintain abstinence for a significant period of time (months) in the past; nevertheless, they are appropriately placed at Level I because they need engagement strategies and intensive case management.

Level II: Intensive Outpatient Treatment/Partial Hospitalization

Level II encompasses intensive outpatient treatment services, which may be delivered in a wide variety of outpatient or partial hospitalization settings. Such treatment may be offered during the day, before or after work or school, in the evening, or on a weekend. For appropriately selected patients, Level II programs provide essential education and treatment services while allowing patients to apply their newly acquired skills in "real world" environments.

Level II treatment programs have the capacity to arrange for medical and psychiatric consultation, psychopharmacological consultation, medication management, and 24-hour crisis services. They provide comprehensive biopsychosocial assessments and individualized treatment plans that are developed in consultation with the patient. Such plans include problem formulation, treatment goals, and measurable treatment objectives. In addition, the programs have active affiliations with other levels of care and can help the patient access support services such as child care, vocational training, and transportation.

Beyond the essential services, many Level II programs provide psychopharmacologic assessment and treatment and have the capacity to effectively treat patients who have complex co-occurring mental and substance-related disorders.

Some programs also can provide overnight housing for patients who have problems related to family environment or transportation but who do not need the supervision or 24-hour access to services afforded by a Level III program. Such structured day and evening treatment programs "unbundle" actual clinical treatment from around-the-clock supervised living environments that include overnight housing.

Treatment Levels Within Level II

Increasingly, distinctions are made among various subtypes of Level II programs. Criteria are offered here for two variations: Intensive Outpatient (Level II.1) and Partial Hospitalization (Level II.5) programs.

Intensive outpatient programs (IOPs) generally provide 9 or more hours of structured programming per week, consisting primarily of counseling and education about substance-related and mental health problems. The patient's needs for psychiatric and medical services are addressed through consultation and referral arrangements if the patient is stable and requires only maintenance monitoring. (Services provided outside the primary program must be tightly coordinated.)

Intensive outpatient treatment differs from partial hospitalization (Level II.5) programs in the intensity of clinical services that are directly available. Specifically, most intensive outpatient programs have less capacity to effectively treat patients who have substantial unstable medical and psychiatric problems than do partial hospitalization programs.

Partial hospitalization programs generally feature 20 or more hours of clinically intensive programming per week, as specified in the patient's treatment plan. Level II.5 partial hospitalization programs typically have direct access to psychiatric, medical, and laboratory services, and thus are better able than Level II.1 programs to meet needs identified in Dimensions 1, 2, and 3, which warrant daily monitoring or management but which can be appropriately addressed in a structured outpatient setting.

Patients who meet Level III criteria in Dimensions 4, 5, or 6 and who otherwise would be placed in a Level III program may be considered for placement in a Level II.5 program if the patient resides in a facility that provides 24-hour support and structure and that limits access to alcohol and other drugs, such as a correctional facility or other licensed health care facility or a supervised living situation.

Length of Service

The duration of treatment varies with the severity of the patient's illness and his or her response to treatment.

Co-Occurring Mental and Substance-Related Disorders

The services of a Level II treatment program are appropriate for patients with co-occurring mental and substance-related disorders if the mental health and addiction treatment services are integrated into the intensive outpatient or partial hospitalization program. Such patients require active mental health services, which should be delivered through Level II.1 Dual Diagnosis Capable or Dual Diagnosis Enhanced programs.

Level III: Residential/Inpatient Treatment

Level III programs offer organized treatment services that feature a planned regimen of care in a 24-hour residential setting. Treatment services adhere to defined policies, procedures, and clinical protocols. They are housed in, or affiliated with, permanent facilities where patients can reside safely. (One of the purposes of these programs is to demonstrate aspects of a positive recovery environment.) They are staffed 24 hours a day. Mutual/self-help group meetings usually are available onsite.

Level III encompasses four types of programs:

- Level III.1: Clinically Managed Low-Intensity Residential Treatment
- Level III.3: Clinically Managed Medium-Intensity Residential Treatment
- Level III.5: Clinically Managed High-Intensity Residential Treatment
- Level III.7: Medically Monitored Inpatient Treatment

The defining characteristic of all Level III programs is that they serve individuals who, because of specific functional deficits, need safe and stable living environments in order to develop their recovery skills. Such living environments may be housed in the same facility as the treatment services, or they may be in separate facilities that are affiliated with the treatment provider. In the latter situation, the relationship between the living environment and the treatment provider must be sufficiently close to allow specific aspects of the individual treatment plan to be addressed in both facilities.

The sublevels within Level III exist on a continuum ranging from the least intensive residential services to the most intensive medically monitored intensive inpatient services. Indeed, Level III always has consisted of a range of intensities of service. The intent never was to create just four discrete sublevels of care within Level III, but rather to create a range of intensities, with each designated sublevel (such as Level III.3) suggesting a particular point within that range. When a program provides Level III services that exceed the intensity usually ascribed to that level, or can appropriately treat an individual who has a more severe illness than usually is addressed at that level, it should be considered an enhanced service.

The term "clinically managed" is used to describe Level III.1 through III.5 programs. Individuals who are appropriately placed in the clinically managed levels of care have minimal problems with intoxication or withdrawal (Dimension 1) and few biomedical complications (Dimension 2), so onsite physician services are not required. Such individuals may have relatively stable problems in Axis I and/or less stable problems in Axis II (Dimension 3) of the *Diagnostic and Statistical Manual of Mental Disorders (DSM)* of the American Psychiatric Association. Many also have significant deficits in the areas of readiness to change (Dimension 4), relapse, continued use or continued problem potential (Dimension 5), or recovery environment (Dimension 6). Therefore, they are in need of interventions directed by appropriately trained and credentialed addiction treatment staff. Such individuals also need case management services to facilitate their reintegration into the larger community.

Length of Service

While the duration of treatment varies with the severity of an individual's illness and his or her response to treatment, the length of service in clinically managed Level III programs tends to be longer than in the more intensive medically monitored and medically managed levels of care.

Some individuals enter Level III programs under a court order that specifies their length of stay. However, treatment professionals have a responsibility to make admission, continued service, and discharge decisions based on their own clinical impressions of an individual's assessed needs and treatment progress. Thus, if a patient has improved sufficiently to warrant discharge or transfer, the treatment professional has a responsibility to contact the appropriate court and seek to have the court order amended.

Co-Occurring Mental and Substance-Related Disorders

Level III programs that treat individuals with co-occurring mental and substance-related disorders typically integrate mental health and addiction treatment services and incorporate mental health professionals into the treatment staff. Such programs generally are more flexible, more individualized and less confrontational than the typical Level III program. There is considerable variation in program activities, as well as in the duration of program stages. The intensity of interpersonal encounters is considerably reduced, reliance on educational and skill-building approaches is increased, and the programs are more closely tailored to address the specific mental and substance-related problems of individual patients. The mental health component of treatment is not focused on intensive psychiatric, medical, or nursing care, but rather on support for reshaping coping skills and mental functioning.

Level IV: Medically Managed Intensive Inpatient Treatment

Level IV medically managed intensive inpatient treatment is an organized service, delivered in an acute care inpatient setting. It is appropriate for patients whose acute biomedical, emotional, behavioral, and cognitive problems are so severe that they require primary medical and nursing care.

Level IV program services are delivered by an interdisciplinary staff of addiction-credentialed physicians and other appropriately credentialed treatment professionals. Such a program encompasses a planned regimen of 24-hour medically directed evaluation and treatment services, provided under a defined set of policies, procedures, and clinical protocols.

Treatment is provided 24 hours a day in a permanent facility with inpatient beds. The full resources of a general acute care or psychiatric hospital are available. Although treatment is specific to substance dependence disorders, the skills of the interdisciplinary team and the availability of support services allow the conjoint treatment of any co-occurring biomedical conditions and mental disorders that need to be addressed.

Length of Service

The duration of treatment varies with the severity of the patient's illness and his or her response to treatment.

Co-Occurring Mental and Substance-Related Disorders

The services of a Level IV program are appropriate for patients who have severe, unstable mental and substance dependence disorders. Such disorders typically require a range of medical, nursing, and other clinical interventions that can be delivered safely only in a 24-hour medically managed setting. They may involve:

- Co-occurring severe substance-related and mental disorders, such as an acutely suicidal patient who also is acutely in need of medical detoxification.
- Severe intoxication or withdrawal problems or other severe biomedical conditions that occur simultaneously with more stabilized mental health problems.
- Severe mental health problems that co-occur with more stabilized substance dependence problems.

Because Level IV program services are the most intensive in the continuum of care, their principal focus is the stabilization of the patient and preparation for his or her transfer to a less intensive setting for continuing care.

DOMAINS FOR ASSESSING RISK IN DIMENSION 5

This Supplement proposes a revised conceptual organization for assessing a patient's risk of relapse, based on a review of the constructs and criteria developed for earlier editions of the ASAM Patient Placement Criteria. (A more comprehensive description can be found in Appendix C of the *ASAM PPC-2*R, pages 341–353.) The revised constructs offer face validity on several levels of basic and clinical research knowledge, including behavioral pharmacology, behavioral psychology, learning theory, and psychopathology, and have been organized into four domains for assessment in Dimension 5.

Developing a multidimensional Risk Profile involves integrating biopsychosocial data from the patient's history and current status into a succinct summary. The four domains described in this chapter—history and pattern of substance use; response to drug effects; response to external stimuli; and cognitive and behavioral measures of temperament, vulnerability, and resilience—offer a conceptually clear *sequence of factors* to use in assessing risk. Each domain is further divided into several subdomains, which contain specific elements of the assessment profile within that domain. Patients are evaluated separately in each domain, after which the results for all the domains are combined in a comprehensive risk assessment and treatment plan.

Domain 1: History and Pattern of Substance Use

This domain includes elements of the problem history, such as duration, severity, and chronicity, as well as response to treatment in the past. *History* may apply to the patient's problems with substance use, abuse, or addiction, or to other aspects of the patient's situation, such as the presence of a co-occurring psychiatric disorder or medical condition. Studies also show that factors such as onset of alcohol or drug problems before age 25, never having lived as married, failure to complete a high school education or GED, and being unemployed all are strong predictors of continued use or relapse. Useful questions include the following:

Subdomain 1a: Duration of Use. The key questions are: "How long has the individual had a problem with alcohol use?" and "At what age did it begin?" The longer the duration of problem drinking and the earlier its onset, the more likely it will continue in the absence of aggressive intervention.

Subdomain 1b: Amount of Use. The key questions are "How much does the individual drink?" and "Has the amount increased over time?" Elements include frequency of drinking (e.g., daily pattern, binge pattern, how many days per week, and the like) and quantity consumed (e.g., how many drinks per occasion or drinking day, how many drinks per week, and the like). Amount is a major component of severity and an essential consideration in developing a treatment plan.

Subdomain 1c: Pattern of Change. The key question is: "How chronic has the problem been; that is, over the course of problematic alcohol use, have there been any meaningful changes, particularly periods of abstinence?" There is a decided difference in risk rating between two patients with similar durations of problem use, where one patient has used alcohol sporadically, with intermittent periods of sobriety, while the other patient has used steadily and without interruption. Such differences are essential considerations in the development of a treatment plan.

Another important component of the patient's history is his or her response to past treatment episodes or other attempts to change. The key questions are: "Has the patient had periods of abstinence and/or improvements in functioning following past treatment episodes?" "How long did those periods last?" "How did the patient achieve those periods of abstinence?" "What methods have and have not been effective?" "What events preceded the patient's relapse to substance use?" Clinical history is a good predictor of future recovery and relapse risk.

Whether or not a patient has experienced formal treatment, the outcome of any past effort to reduce or stop substance use can provide useful information, even if it involves a substance other than the one that is the current primary concern (e.g., it may be helpful to know if the patient has successfully quit smoking) or how well the patient has managed other chronic disorders (e.g., diabetes or hypertension). Previous positive response (or lack of response) to other external influences or changes in life circumstances also may be predictive.

Domain 2: Response to Substance Effects

This domain encompasses both positive and negative reinforcement. Factors to consider include the following:

Subdomain 2a: Positive Reinforcement (or Reward Craving). The key factor is the degree to which the patient anticipates pleasure or euphoria as a result of his or her substance use. The key questions include: "Does the patient get pleasure or a 'boost' from using? What does the patient enjoy from about using?" "Does the patient experience a 'hunger' for using?"

Subdomain 2b: Negative Reinforcement (or Relief Craving). The key factor is the degree to which the patient anticipates relief of discomfort as a result of his or her substance use. Note that negative reinforcement is not used here to describe *actual* symptoms of withdrawal or abstinence (which are addressed in Dimension 1, Intoxication/Withdrawal), but rather the patient's *expectations* of the relief of withdrawal or unpleasant experiences during abstinence. Many patients describe alcohol use as providing relief from stress or worries or dysphoric mood states or report that such use makes them feel "normal." The key questions are: "Does the patient get relief from negative experiences by using?" "Does the patient anticipate or fear symptoms such as insomnia, agitation, anxiety, inability to cope, and the like when they stop using?" "Does the patient desire alcohol to relieve negative feelings or symptoms that emerge when they stop drinking?"

Domain 3: Response to External Stimuli

This domain includes both acute cues and chronic stressors. Factors to consider include the following:

Subdomain 3a: Response to cues or triggers, such as alcohol advertising or being in the presence of others who are drinking or using drugs.

Subdomain 3b: Response to acute and/or chronic stressors, such as social pressures or conflicts, as well as ongoing environmental challenges such as homelessness, divorce, or financial problems. Table 6-1 provides examples of potential stressors that can be used as part of an assessment inventory.

Domain 4: Cognitive and Behavioral Measures of Temperament, Vulnerability, and Resilience

This domain encompasses coping skills, impulsivity, locus of control, and passive or passive-aggressive behaviors also are important indicators. Factors to consider include the following:

Subdomain 4a: Locus of Control and Self-Efficacy. The key question is whether the patient has an internal sense of self-determination and confidence that he or she can direct his or her own behavioral change.

Subdomain 4b: Coping skills, including stimulus control and other cognitive strategies.

Subdomain 4c: Impulsivity. This includes dimensional traits of risk-taking and thrill- or novelty-seeking, rather than diagnostic categories of psychopathology, which would be assessed in Dimension 3 (although there certainly could be overlap).

Subdomain 4d: Passive and Passive-Aggressive Behavior. The key question is: "Does the individual demonstrate active efforts to anticipate and cope with internal and external stressors, or does he or she abdicate responsibility or assign it to others?" Note that these are personality traits rather than pathological conditions, which are assessed in Dimension 3.

USING THE MATRIX TO DEVELOP A RISK PROFILE

To use the Matrix most effectively, the clinician performs a comprehensive assessment of the patient's strengths and problems in each of six dimensions. Once a problem list is created, it is prioritized by severity (e.g., Dimension 2, advanced liver disease in an alcohol-dependent patient), risk (as in Dimension 3, suicidal thought with high lethality), or interference (reflected

TABLE 6-1

Inventory of Relapse Stressors and Environmental Problems

(Non-italicized material is from the DSM-IV, Axis IV. Italicized material represents a consensus of experienced addiction professionals.)

Problems with primary support group (check all that apply)

___ Death of a family member
___ Health problems in the family
___ Disruption of family by separation, divorce, or estrangement
___ Removal from the home
___ Remarriage of a parent
___ Sexual, *emotional*, or physical abuse
___ Parental overprotection
___ Neglect of child
___ Inadequate discipline
___ Discord with siblings
___ Birth of a sibling
___ *Acting out children*
___ *Single parent, recent blended family*
___ *Significant other an active substance abuser or dependent*
___ *Significant other threatened by recovery or not supportive of recovery efforts*
___ *Significant other a using partner and/or dealer*
___ *Absence of a positive primary social support system*
___ *Threatened removal of a child by the state child protective agency*

Problems related to the social environment (check all that apply)

___ Death or loss of friend
___ Inadequate social support
___ Living alone
___ Difficulty with acculturation
___ Discrimination
___ Adjustment to lifestyle transition (such as retirement)
___ *Social support system populated by other substance-using, -abusing or -dealing individuals*
___ *Absence of a positive (non-using) social support system*
___ *Living with an active addict*
___ *Living with a dealer*
___ *Rampant drug use/sale in neighborhood*
___ *Rampant drug use/sale at work site/school*
___ *Pressure to use substances by other employees/students*
___ *Employer not supportive of recovery efforts*
___ *Impending deployment (military)*

Educational problems (check all that apply)

___ Illiteracy; academic problems
___ Discord with teachers or classmates
___ Inadequate school environment
___ *Absence of high school diploma or GED*

Occupational problems (check all that apply)

___ Unemployment, threat of job loss
___ Stressful work schedule
___ Difficult work conditions

___ Job dissatisfaction
___ Job change
___ Conflict with boss or co-workers
___ *Lack of vocational skills*
___ *Lack of job opportunity*
___ *Lack of experience acquiring and maintaining employment*
___ *Employment associated with ready access to psychoactive substances (bartenders; health care professionals)*
___ *Inadequate transportation (lack of public transportation, no reliable car, no valid driver's license)*
___ *Lack of child care*
___ *Felony conviction or other criminal record*
___ *On parole or probation*
Housing problems (check all that apply)
___ Homelessness
___ Inadequate housing
___ Unsafe housing/neighborhood
___ Discord with neighbors or landlord
___ *Psychoactive substance availability in housing (beer machines in military barracks; drinking in college dormitories)*
___ *Housing situation features widespread substance use (public housing)*
___ *Inadequate income for housing*
Economic problems (check all that apply)
___ Extreme poverty, inadequate finances
___ Insufficient welfare support
___ *Dealing drugs is primary way to make money*
___ *Money owed to dealers*
___ *Unable to acquire psychotropic medications because of inadequate financial resources*
Problems with access to health care services (check all that apply)
___ Inadequate health care services
___ Transportation to health care services unavailable
___ Inadequate/absent health care insurance
___ *Inadequate or absent public funding for addiction treatment services*
___ *Recent loss of health care benefits (e.g., loss of Medicaid coverage when moving from welfare to work)*
___ *Absence of the appropriate level or type of addiction services*
Problems related to interaction with the legal system/crime (check all that apply)
___ Arrest
___ Incarceration
___ Litigation
___ Victim of crime
___ *Upcoming trial*
___ *Threat of incarceration for past crimes*
___ *On probation or parol*
Other psychosocial and environmental problems (check all that apply)
___ Exposure to disasters, war, other hostilities
___ Discord with nonfamily care givers such as counselor, social worker or physician
___ Unavailability of social service agencies
___ *Transportation problems*
___ *Child care problems*
___ *Emotional or behavioral conditions that are likely to be worsened by stressor*

in Dimension 6, lack of child care or transportation for a patient who appears to be a likely candidate for an outpatient level of care).

In column 1 of the Matrix, each of the prioritized problems is assigned a Risk Rating, ranging from 0 (no or stable problem), to 1 (minimal risk), 2 (moderate risk), 3 (significant risk), or 4 (severe risk). Based on the Risk Rating assigned in column 1, the appropriate services are selected from column 2, as are the modalities for delivering the services, and the intensity/level of care are selected from column 3. For example, if a patient is assessed as being at significant risk for relapse to alcohol use (Dimension 5, Risk Rating 3) in column 1, the services selected from column 2 might include relapse prevention treatment services such as individual and group counseling, as well as initiation of a medication for alcohol dependence (modalities). In column 3, placement at a particular level of care is determined. It is not unusual for particular service needs and intensities to be met at more than one level of care. Patients should be placed at the least intensive level at which the patient can safely and effectively receive treatment.

Table 6-2 demonstrates how the severity of relapse risk is reflected in the various domains. The examples describe patient characteristics in each domain at ascending levels of risk, as a guide to determining a Risk Rating. Once a Risk Rating has been determined, the Dimension 5 Matrix on pages 112–117 can be used to determine the patient's service needs and level of care.

CORE TREATMENT INTERVENTIONS IN DIMENSION 5

Table 6-3 is a guide to matching available treatment interventions to the patient's assessed needs in Dimension 5. Patients may benefit from a variety of relapse prevention interventions, and the appropriate selection is a matter of clinical judgment. Patients who are at lower levels of risk generally benefit from a smaller number of targeted interventions, while those at higher levels of risk typically need a greater number of coordinated interventions.

Note that the table is a representative but not exhaustive listing, and interventions and strategies not listed here also may be appropriate if supported by research and/or clinical consensus. See the Guide to Determining Risk Ratings in Dimension 5 (pages 112–117) to determine the patient's Risk Rating, and the Dimension 5 Matrix (pages 112–117) for a guide to matching interventions and level of care to the patient's assessed needs.

RISK ASSESSMENT MATRIX FOR DIMENSION 5

In each assessment dimension (which correspond to Dimensions 1 to 6 of the ASAM Patient Placement Criteria), the Risk Rating (first column of the Matrix) suggest the severity of the patient's problem in that dimension. The treatment priorities represented by the Service Needs and Interventions (second column of the Matrix) suggest the specific types of treatment services/modalities the patient requires to appropriately address his or her multidimensional service needs. The Level of Care and Setting (third column of the Matrix) in turn suggests the intensity and resources with which those services should be effectively delivered within a range of settings and levels of care.

TABLE 6-2

Assessing Severity of Relapse Risk in Each Domain

Risk Rating = 0

A Risk Rating of **0** indicates that the patient is at minimal or no observable risk for substance-related problems. Such a patient typically is stable and has good coping skills. The following describe a patient with a Risk Rating of 0:

Domain 1: History and Pattern of Substance Use

- The patient has a history and pattern of substance use that is marked by negligible chronicity and severity (or, if high severity, the patient has been abstinent for an extended period of time, with significantly improved functioning).
- The patient evidences an extremely positive response to treatment or other influences (e.g., the patient has been abstinent for an extended period of time, with significantly improved functioning and sense of well-being).

Domain 2: Response to Substance Effects

- The patient derives negligible reward or pleasure derived from substance use (e.g., the most recent period of use provided no reinforcement for continued use).
- The patient's motive for use of substances is not to avoid or relieve the discomfort of acute or subacute withdrawal. He or she expresses no concern about discomfort or bad feelings if substance use is interrupted or stopped.

Domain 3: Response to External Stimuli

- The patient does not react to cues and is minimally troubled by substance-related cues and triggers.
- The patient does not react with instability to stress, and is minimally troubled by acute or persistent stressors.

Domain 4: Cognitive and Behavioral Measures of Temperament, Vulnerabilities, and Resilience

- The patient has a strong sense of self-determination and confidence in his or her ability to direct change. His or her behavior is self-directed.
- The patient has excellent coping skills. He or she deals effectively with challenges and adversity.
- The patient exhibits minimal impulsivity. He or she does not engage in risk-taking or problematic thrill-seeking behaviors and is deliberate and thoughtful in reactions.
- The patient does not exhibit passive or passive-aggressive behavior. The patient takes charge of efforts to manage resources and stressors, and accepts responsibility for his or her actions.

Risk Rating = 1

A Risk Rating of **1** indicates that the patient is at *mild* risk for continuation of or relapse to substance use. The following describes a patient with a Risk Rating of 1:

Domain 1: History and Pattern of Substance Use

- The patient has a history and pattern of substance use that is marked by mild chronicity and severity (e.g., a brief period of use, followed by a period with markedly improving functioning and sense of well-being).
- The patient evidences a strongly positive response to treatment or other influences (e.g., he or she has been abstinent for a long enough period to have achieved improved functioning).

Domain 2: Response to Substance Effects

- The patient derives mild reward or pleasure from substance use (e.g., the most recent period of use provided little reinforcement for continued use).

(continues)

TABLE 6-2 *(continued)*

Assessing Severity of Relapse Risk in Each Domain

- The patient is somewhat likely to use substances to avoid or relieve the discomfort of withdrawal (acute or subacute), and expresses some concern about discomfort or bad feelings if substance use is interrupted or stopped.

Domain 3: Response to External Stimuli

- The patient has mild reaction to cues, and a mild response to trigger objects or situations.
- The patient has mild reaction to acute or persistent stressors.

Domain 4: Cognitive and Behavioral Measures of Temperament, Vulnerabilities, and Resilience

- The patient has a generally consistent sense of self-determination and confidence in his or her ability to direct change, but with behavior that is still negatively affected by external triggers.
- The patient demonstrates generally consistent coping skills. However, he or she appears to have some difficulty in dealing effectively with challenges and adversity.
- The patient evidences mild impulsivity. He or she engages in a low level of risk-taking or thrill-seeking behaviors.
- The patient exhibits mildly passive or passive-aggressive behaviors. He or she is only mildly or inconsistently active in taking charge of efforts to manage resources and stressors, and generally accepts responsibility for his or her actions.

Risk Rating = 2

A Risk Rating of 2 indicates that the patient is at *moderate* risk for continuation of or relapse to substance use. The following describes a patient with a Risk Rating of 2:

Domain 1: History and Pattern of Substance Use

- The patient exhibits some (but inadequately consistent) response to past treatment episodes or other influences. The response seems likely to be reinitiated and sustained.

Domain 2: Response to Substance Effects

- The patient derives moderate reward or pleasure from substance use (e.g., the most recent period of use provided little reinforcement for continued use).
- The patient is likely to use substances to avoid or relieve the discomfort of withdrawal (acute or subacute), and expresses concern about discomfort or bad feelings if substance use is interrupted or stopped.

Domain 3: Response to External Stimuli

- The patient has a moderate reaction to cues, and a moderate response to trigger objects or situations.
- The patient is moderately troubled and destabilized by acute or persistent stressors.

Domain 4: Cognitive and Behavioral Measures of Temperament, Vulnerabilities, and Resilience

- The patient has a history and pattern of substance use that is marked by moderate chronicity (duration) or severity.
- The patient has an inconsistent sense of self-determination and confidence in his or her ability to direct change, with behavior that is negatively affected by external triggers.
- The patient demonstrates inconsistent coping skills. The patient has difficulty dealing effectively with challenges and adversity.
- The patient evidences moderate impulsivity. The patient engages in a moderate level of risk-taking or thrill-seeking behaviors.
- The patient exhibits moderately passive or passive-aggressive behavior. The patient is only moderately or inconsistently active in taking charge of efforts to manage resources and stressors, and generally accepts responsibility for his or her actions.

Risk Rating = 3

A Risk Rating of **3** indicates that the patient is at significant risk of relapse or continuation of substance use, but does *not* pose an imminent danger to self or other. Such a patient typically has a long history of substance use, with high severity and possibly chronicity, and may not have responded favorably to previous attempts at intervention. For example, repeated treatment episodes may have had little positive effect on the patient's functioning. He or she may lack the skills to cope with and interrupt his or her substance use or to prevent or limit relapse. The following describes a patient with a Risk Rating of 3:

Domain 1: History and Pattern of Substance Use

- The patient has a history and pattern of substance use marked by significant chronicity and severity, with a long history of use and/or repeated unsuccessful or unsustained attempts at abstinence.
- The patient demonstrates a poor response to change induced by treatment or other influences (e.g., he or she has been abstinent only for short periods of time, with little improvement in functioning).

Domain 2: Response to Substance Effects

- The patient derives intense reward or pleasure from substance use (e.g., the most recent period of use provided very strong reinforcement for continued use).
- The patient is very likely to continue or relapse to substance use to avoid or relieve the discomfort of withdrawal, and/or expresses significant concern about discomfort or bad feelings if substance use is interrupted or stopped.

Domain 3: Response to External Stimuli

- The patient has a significant reaction to cues, and a strong response to trigger objects or situations.
- The patient has a significant response to stressors.

Domain 4: Cognitive and Behavioral Measures of Temperament, Vulnerabilities, and Resilience

- The patient has a minimal sense of self-determination and confidence, or is unrealistically overconfident, in his or her ability to direct change. The patient's behavior appears to be significantly affected by external triggers.
- The patient exhibits poor coping skills and significant difficulty in dealing effectively with challenges and adversity (negative events typically lead to use).
- The patient has a high level of impulsivity. The patient engages in dangerous risk-taking or thrill-seeking behaviors.
- The patient exhibits passive or passive-aggressive behavior. The patient makes minimal effort to manage resources and stressors, and often abdicates responsibility for his or her actions.

Risk Rating = 4

The patient with a Risk Rating of **4** is at very high risk for relapse. Such a patient lacks the skills to arrest his or her substance use. *The risk of relapse or continued use is such that the patient poses an imminent danger to self and others.* For example, the patient's continued substance use may leads to impulsive, psychotic, or aggressive behaviors. The following describes a patient with a Risk Rating of 4:

Domain 1: History and Pattern of Substance Use

- The patient has a history and pattern of substance use marked by extreme chronicity and severity, with a long history of use and/or repeated unsuccessful or unsustained attempts at abstinence.
- The patient has a negligible response to change induced by treatment or other influences (e.g., the patient has been abstinent only for short periods of time, with little improvement in functioning).
- Relapse or continued use poses an imminent danger to self and/or others.

(continues)

TABLE 6-2 *(continued)*

Assessing Severity of Relapse Risk in Each Domain

Domain 2: Response to Substance Effects

- The patient derives intense reward or pleasure from substance use (e.g., the most recent period of use provided very strong reinforcement for continued use).
- The patient is almost certain to continue or relapse to substance use to avoid or relieve the discomfort of withdrawal, and appears to be intensely concerned about discomfort or bad feelings if substance use is interrupted or stopped.
- Relapse or continued use poses an imminent danger to self and/or others.

Domain 3: Response to External Stimuli

- The patient has an intense reaction to cues, and a very strong response to trigger objects or situations.
- The patient has an intense response to persistent stressors.
- Relapse or continued use poses an imminent danger to self and/or others.

Domain 4: Cognitive and Behavioral Measures of Temperament, Vulnerabilities, and Resilience

- The patient exhibits inappropriate overconfidence or undue pessimism about his or her ability to direct change. The patient's behavior is almost entirely governed by external triggers.
- The patient has poor coping skills. The patient has significant difficulty in dealing effectively with challenges and adversity. Negative events consistently lead to us.
- The patient has a very high level of impulsivity. The patient engages in dangerous risk-taking or thrill-seeking behaviors.
- The patient exhibits consistently passive or passive-aggressive behavior. The patient is unable to take charge of efforts to manage resources and stressors, and consistently abdicates responsibility for his or her behavior.
- Relapse or continued use poses an imminent danger to self and/or others.

TABLE 6-3

Core Interventions in Dimension 5 Domains: Indicators of Severity and Risk with Corresponding Pharmacologic and Nonpharmacologic Therapies

Indicators of Severity and Risk	Relevant Pharmacologic and Nonpharmacologic Therapies
DOMAIN 1: HISTORY AND PATTERN OF SUBSTANCE USE	
Indicators of Risk	**Possible Interventions**
If the patient's substance use history is chronic and/or severe (as indicated by pattern, duration, and amount), consider the following approaches:	• Initiate a broad array of multiple, simultaneous relapse prevention interventions. • Initiate pharmacotherapy with an antiaddiction medication (especially if the patient relapsed or was unable to stop alcohol use after earlier treatment without medication support). • If the patient has a strong family history of alcoholism, consider naltrexone (in either the oral or extended-release injectable formulation).

Indicators of Severity and Risk	Relevant Pharmacologic and Nonpharmacologic Therapies
If the patient responded positively to previous attempts to change (through treatment or other influences), consider the following approaches:	• Work with the patient to identify what was helpful in the past and reinitiate or reapply those strategies. • Add one or more novel element(s) or approach(es) to the previously successful treatment plan to increase its long-term effectiveness. • Add more leverage or contingency management to the previously successful treatment plan to increase its long-term effectiveness.
If the patient had a poor response to previous attempts to change (through treatment or other influences), consider the following approaches:	• Add additional maintenance phase monitoring and/or interventions to the previously successful treatment plan to increase its sustainability. • Attempt to identify past barriers to effectiveness and devise strategies to address them. • Implement a novel treatment plan or approach, or serial revisions to the existing treatment plan. • Add more leverage or contingency management to the treatment plan to increase its effectiveness. • Add systems incentives to consolidate the patient's engagement in treatment, or increase the duration of treatment. • Initiate or reintroduce pharmacotherapy with an antiaddiction medication, especially if the patient has relapsed or has been unable to stop alcohol use without medication support. • If the patient already is taking an antiaddiction medication, modify the therapeutic regimen (e.g., by switching to a different medication, or taking steps to enhance medication adherence/compliance).
DOMAIN 2: RESPONSE TO SUBSTANCE EFFECTS	
Indicators of Risk	**Possible Interventions**
If the patient's history reflects the influence of *positive reinforcement* (i.e., deriving significant reward or pleasure from drinking), and/or the patient is experiencing subjective craving, consider the following approaches:	• Acknowledge the pleasure the patient derives from alcohol and the feelings of loss that may attend giving it up. • Identify alternative activities that provide pleasure or reward. • Help the patient conduct a functional analysis of the pros and cons of alcohol use (e.g., a decisional balance exercise). • If the patient has cravings for alcohol or anticipates pleasure from drinking, consider naltrexone (in either the oral or extended-release injectable formulation).
If the patient's history reflects the influence of *negative reinforcement* (i.e., drinking to avoid or relieve the discomfort of discontinuation or withdrawal, acute or subacute), consider the following approaches:	• Help the patient conduct a functional analysis of the pros and cons of alcohol use (e.g., a decisional balance exercise). • If the patient has a history of significant physiologic symptoms ac companying withdrawal from alcohol, consider acamprosate. • If the patient anticipates unpleasant consequences (e.g., anxiety, dysphoria, discomfort, etc.) on cessation of alcohol use, or the relief of such symptoms through resumption of drinking, identify distraction techniques or relaxation/ stress relief activities, and consider acamprosate.

(continues)

TABLE 6-3 ***(continued)***

Core Interventions in Dimension 5 Domains: Indicators of Severity and Risk with Corresponding Pharmacologic and Nonpharmacologic Therapies

Indicators of Severity and Risk	Relevant Pharmacologic and Nonpharmacologic Therapies
	• If the patient would likely avoid drinking if there were more concrete, immediate, and predictable consequences (especially if the patient has the goal of abstinence and has no more than moderate impulsivity), consider disulfiram in combination with suitable adherence/compliance enhancement measures. • If the patient experiences persistent negative affective symptoms (such as anxiety, depression, dysphoria, or anhedonia) on cessation of alcohol use, consider psychiatric evaluation for a mood disorder.
DOMAIN 3: RESPONSE TO EXTERNAL STIMULI	
Indicators of Risk	**Possible Interventions**
If the patient has a significant reaction to external cues and triggers (objects and/or situations), consider the following approaches:	• Cue desensitization therapy. • Cognitive–behavioral therapy (CBT), with an emphasis on stimulus control and avoidance. • Strategies to moderate the effects of or remove the patient from the cue-filled environment. • Avoidance of negative peer contamination. • Development of pro-social peer supports.
If the patient is strongly reactive to acute or chronic stress, consider the following approaches:	• Relaxation training. • Strategies to moderate the effects of or remove the patient from a toxic or stress-filled environment. • Addressing identified stressors. • Helping the patient access relevant supports. • If the patient is significantly destabilized by stressors, consider the possibility that the patient has co-occurring depression or another psychiatric disorder, which should be addressed through referral for a psychiatric assessment.
DOMAIN 4: COGNITIVE AND BEHAVIORAL MEASURES OF TEMPERAMENT, VULNERABILITIES, AND RESILIENCE	
Indicators of Risk	**Possible Interventions**
If the patient exhibits destabilizing vulnerabilities of temperament, consider the following approaches:	• Encourage self-knowledge through a review of personal assets and vulnerabilities in response to specific situations.

Indicators of Severity and Risk	Relevant Pharmacologic and Nonpharmacologic Therapies
If the patient demonstrates unstably extroverted traits (Cluster B), which may lead to stress reactions that are over-intense or catastrophic compared to normal reactions, consider the following approaches:	• Orient the patient toward an emphasis on behavioral change and deemphasize his or her preoccupation with feelings. • Use therapies that teach self-regulation of affect, such as Dialectical Behavior Therapy (DBT) or similar approaches.
If the patient evidences problems with self-determination, self-efficacy, external locus of control, and/or poor confidence in ability to direct change, consider the following approaches:	• Employ strategies to enhance the patient's adherence to the treatment plan. • Emphasize external influences and motivators (e.g., criminal justice leverage, contingency management, and the like.) • Increase the frequency of monitoring, combined with use of proximal goals focused on treatment service utilization. • Take steps to engage the patient in a positive social support system such as AA, a therapeutic community, or supportive living arrangement (halfway house, recovery house, etc.). • Help the patient find nonprofessional peer support (as through an AA sponsor, recovery mentorship, peer-to-peer recovery assistance, network therapy, and the like).
If the patient evidences problems with poor coping skills and difficulty in dealing effectively with challenges and adversity, consider the following approaches:	• Emphasize practical, solution-focused approaches. • Examine the degree to which the patient's drinking represents an effort to overcome specific deficits in coping skills (such as anxiety associated with social phobias, recurrent conflicts, or characteristic predicaments) and address those deficits.
If the patient exhibits problems with impulsivity and/or engaging in high levels of risk-taking or thrill-seeking behaviors, consider the following approaches:	• Emphasize external supports and monitoring. • Employ strategies to enhance the patient's adherence to the treatment plan. • Help the patient avoid negative peer contamination and find pro-social peer supports. • For risk-taking or thrill-seeking behaviors, encourage high-intensity or high-excitement pro-social leisure activities as safer alternatives.
If the patient exhibits problems with passive or passive-aggressive approaches, inability to take charge of efforts to manage resources and stressors, or abdication of responsibility for actions, consider the following approaches:	• Employ strategies to enhance the patient's adherence to the treatment plan. • Agree on clear short-term behavioral goals. • Encourage the patient to pursue affiliations with potential helpers such as sober, pro-social peers or family. • Encourage the patient to join self-help or mutual-help groups. • Provide assertiveness training.
If the patient's social support system is weak or absent, consider the following approaches:	• Encourage the patient to reach out to underutilized potential supports such as family, friends, coworkers, or peers. • Help the patient link to a positive social support system such as AA, Oxford House, a faith community, and the like.

MATRIX FOR DIMENSION 5: RELAPSE PREVENTION

The patient's assessed needs should be considered in each ASAM Dimension. The interaction between Dimension 5 and other Dimensions may increase or reduce assessed severity (see the discussion of Dimensional interactions in Chapter 1).

RISK RATING	SERVICE NEEDS AND INTERVENTIONS	LEVEL OF CARE AND SETTING
General Considerations Considerations and services that are common to all risk levels are described here. The sections that follow identify issues and services that have particular relevance to or urgency for patients with specific Risk Ratings.	**Service Needs** Patients may benefit from a variety of relapse prevention interventions (*see the discussions in Chapters 4 and 5, particularly the list of core interventions in Table 6-3, as well as Appendix B*). Patients who are at lower levels of risk generally benefit from a smaller number of targeted interventions, while those at higher levels of risk typically need a larger number of coordinated interventions. **Treatment Interventions** If treatment has included a pharmacotherapy, the patient should be encouraged to continue it as supervised maintenance treatment until the patient and physician agree to attempt monitored discontinuation. At present, there is no clear evidence to indicate an optimal duration of maintenance treatment. However, there is some emerging clinical consensus that pharmacotherapy should be continued for at least one year past the point of sustained abstinence.	**Coordination of Services** Addiction treatment programs should develop referral relationships with and linkages to addiction medicine specialists who are experienced in evaluating patients and using pharmacotherapies to treat alcohol dependence, so that these services are readily accessible as needed. Any pharmacotherapy should be carefully integrated into the overall treatment plan. When medication management and other addiction treatment services are delivered by separate providers, coordination is vital. **Staffing** Patients who are treated with an antiaddiction medication need frequent initial monitoring and ongoing medication management. This can be performed by an appropriately trained and experienced primary care physician or a specialist in addiction medicine or addiction psychiatry. Addiction counselors involved in the care of patients with alcohol dependence should be aware of the goals of pharmacotherapy and prepared to collaborate in monitoring and supporting it. Treatment programs should have mechanisms in place (such as training and supervision) to foster and support such collaboration.
Risk Rating = 0 (Minimal or no risk) A Risk Rating of **0** indicates that the patient is at *minimal or no observable risk* for substance-related problems in Dimen-	**Service Needs** A Risk Rating of **0** indicates *minimal or no need* for professional treatment services in Dimension 5. Only maintenance services or activities may be needed. **Treatment Interventions** At this level of risk, there is no need to initiate professional services specifically to address problems in Dimension 5. However, the patient may be receiving (and should continue to receive) ongoing maintenance treatment or continuing care.	**Level of Care** The patient with a Risk Rating of **0** who needs maintenance treatment should be placed in a Level I outpatient service. **Setting and Service Delivery** Care can be delivered in an organized outpatient addiction treatment program, a mental health program with an addiction treatment capability, or by an individual practitioner who has the requisite addiction treatment knowledge and skills. Maintenance pharmacotherapy can be provided by an appropriately

sion 5 (*see the guide to the determination of risk ratings*). Such a patient typically is stable and has good coping skills.	If successful treatment in the past has included a pharmacotherapy, the patient should be encouraged to continue such therapy through supervised maintenance treatment until the physician and patient agree to attempt monitored discontinuation. At present, there is no clear evidence as to the optimal duration of maintenance treatment. However, there is some emerging clinical consensus that pharmacotherapy should be continued for at least 12 months past the point of sustained abstinence.	experienced primary care physician or a specialist in addiction medicine or addiction psychiatry.
Risk Rating = 1 (Mild risk) A Risk Rating of 1 indicates that the patient is at *mild risk* for relapse to or continuation of substance use (*see the guide to the determination of risk ratings*). Such a patient typically has fair self-management skills. For example, the patient may have a pattern of harmful drinking or alcohol abuse, but may not meet the criteria for active alcohol dependence. Or the patient *does* meet criteria for alcohol dependence based on a previous pattern of severity and is now experiencing less severe relapse symptoms, following a period of stabilization or improvement.	**Service Needs** A Risk Rating of 1 indicates a need for professional services in Dimension 5. The goal should be to reduce relapse risk by reinforcing the patient's coping skills. For example, if the patient does not have a chronic history or severe pattern of substance use, services may be provided until the patient can be integrated into continuing care or a self- or mutual-help or other nonprofessional group, or a religious or spiritual support community. **Treatment Interventions** The patient with a Risk Rating of 1 may benefit from a variety of relapse prevention interventions (*see the discussions in Chapters 4 and 5, particularly the list of core interventions in Table 6-3, as well as Appendix B*). At this level of risk, a targeted selection of interventions generally provides an appropriate balance between efficacy and patient burden. Such interventions generally are delivered at a low level of intensity. Patients should be educated about all appropriate treatment options, including the availability of antiaddiction medications as a potential addition to the treatment plan in the future, if such medications are needed if previously successful treatment has included pharmacotherapy, the patient should be encouraged to continue or resume it. Initiation of treatment with an antiaddiction medication should be considered if relapse or continued use poses a high risk of potential adverse effects because of severity in other dimensions. The patient also may need recovery support services, such as help with transportation and assistance in meeting the cost of treatment.	**Level of Care** The patient with a Risk Rating of 1 should be placed in a Level I outpatient service. **Setting and Service Delivery** Care can be delivered in an organized outpatient addiction treatment program, a mental health program with an addiction treatment capability, or by an individual practitioner who has the requisite addiction treatment knowledge and skills. Pharmacotherapy can be provided by an appropriately experienced primary care physician or a specialist in addiction medicine or addiction psychiatry. Addiction treatment programs that do not provide their own medical services should develop referral relationships with and linkages to addiction medicine specialists who are experienced in evaluating patients and using pharmacotherapies to treat alcohol dependence. When medication management and other addiction treatment services are delivered by separate providers, coordination is vital.

(*continues*)

RISK RATING	SERVICE NEEDS AND INTERVENTIONS	LEVEL OF CARE AND SETTING
Risk Rating = 2 (Moderate risk) The patient with a Risk Rating of **2** is at *moderate risk* for relapse to or continuation of substance use (*see the guide to the determination of risk ratings*). Such a patient typically exhibits impaired recognition and understanding of substance use relapse issues, but is able to self-manage with prompting. For example, such a patient is externally oriented and tends to blame family or friends, circumstances, or bad luck for his or her relapse or continued use. However, with counseling and encouragement to reach out to an AA sponsor or to attend a SMART recovery group (or a similar support), the patient should be able to improve his or her self-management of urges to use.	**Service Needs** A Risk Rating of **2** indicates a need for specific professional services in Dimension 5 to provide the supports and interventions that will reinforce the patient's self-management skills. Without such interventions, the patient's risk level can escalate quickly. **Treatment Interventions** The patients with a Risk Rating of **2** may benefit from a variety of relapse prevention interventions (*see the discussions in Chapters 4 and 5, particularly the list of core interventions in Table 6-3, as well as Appendix B*). At this level of risk, clinical interventions generally are delivered at a moderate level of intensity. In the absence of contraindications, treatment with an antiaddiction medication should be considered, especially if relapse or continued use poses a high risk of potential adverse effects because of severity in other Dimensions, or if the patient relapsed after earlier treatment without medication support. Services also should include exploration of systems incentives to consolidate the patient's engagement in treatment. (This is an important consideration because of the potential consequences of relapse or continued use.) A patient at this level of risk requires encouragement, guidance, and frequent programmatic supports to improve self-management of urges to use. The patient also may need motivational strategies, structured coping skills, intensive case management and community outreach, assistance in finding supportive living arrangements, and/or assertive community treatment (ACT) (*see the discussions in Chapters 4 and 5, as well as Appendix B*). The patient may need recovery support services, such as help with employment or obtaining educational, child care, and transportation services.	**Level of Care** The patient with a Risk Rating of **2** should be placed in a Level II.1 or II.5 outpatient service. **Setting and Service Delivery** Care can be delivered in an organized outpatient addiction treatment program or a mental health program with an addiction treatment capability. Pharmacotherapy can be provided by an appropriately experienced primary care physician or a specialist in addiction medicine or addiction psychiatry. Addiction treatment programs that treat patients with alcohol dependence of moderate severity should develop the capacity for coordination of care with addiction medicine specialists who can evaluate patients and prescribe pharmacotherapies. Such services should be accessed either through direct availability of addiction medicine services within the program, or close linkages to such services, to facilitate access.
Risk Rating = 3 (Significant risk) The patient with a Risk Rating of **3** is at *significant risk* for relapse to or continuation of substance use (*see the guide to the determination of risk ratings*). Such a patient typically demonstrates little recognition or understanding of	**Service Needs** A Risk Rating of **3** indicates an urgent need for professional services specifically to address the patient's problems in Dimension 5. Because the patient with a Risk Rating of **3** does not pose an imminent danger to self or others, there is not necessarily a need for containment in Dimension 5. However, the level of severity in other dimensions could require stabilization in a 24-hour setting (*see the Interdimensional Severity chart in Chapter 1*). For example, if the patient does not have family or significant others who can provide appropriate 24-hour structure and supervision, such support may be found in a supportive living	**Level of Care** The patient with a Risk Rating of **3** should be placed at a level of care and in a setting that provides services at a level of intensity that corresponds to the patient's readiness to change and ability to utilize the services offered. In some situations, residential/inpatient monitoring (sometimes as a step-down from a detoxification or supervised withdrawal level of care or as a step up from a less intensive level of care) may be necessary to establish the lead-in period of abstinence recommended before pharmacotherapy with an antiaddiction medication is initiated.

<table>
<tr>
<td>relapse issues and has poor skills to cope with and interrupt substance-related problems or to avoid or limit relapse.

Repeated treatment episodes may have had little positive effect on the patient's functioning. Such a patient typically has an extensive history of use, marked by high levels of severity and possibly chronicity, and may not have responded favorably to previous attempts at intervention. He or she may lack the skills to cope with and interrupt his or her substance use problem or to prevent or limit relapse.

For example, the patient may leave a medically supervised withdrawal program early and against medical advice; or may be passive about attending self- or mutual-help groups, in the belief that he or she does not need supports for recovery.

However, such a patient does not pose an imminent danger to self or others and is able to care for himself or herself. For example, the patient may have undergone repeated episodes of medically supervised withdrawal and may be unable to cope with recurring</td>
<td>arrangement or treatment setting. If the patient is physically dependent and at risk for severe withdrawal, supervised detoxification/withdrawal in a 24-hour setting is strongly recommended (refer to Dimension 1). If the patient is homeless or does not have a supportive living environment, placement in a 24-hour-support setting may be appropriate (refer to Dimension 6).

Treatment Interventions

High-intensity relapse prevention services are urgently needed and should be offered promptly (see the discussions in Chapters 4 and 5, particularly the list of core interventions in Table 6-3, as well as Appendix B).

Patients at higher levels of risk typically need a broader array of multiple, simultaneous interventions. Such patients typically need help with compliance/adherence to the various components of the treatment regimen, including pharmacotherapies.

The patient with a Risk Rating of 3 may have failed previous interventions and should be offered new treatment modalities and adjunctive therapies as part of a comprehensive treatment plan. In the absence of contraindications, initiation of treatment with an antiaddiction medication should be strongly considered. Pharmacotherapies should be routinely available as a component of treatment for patients with a Risk Rating of 3.

The patient also may need motivational strategies, structured coping skills, intensive case management and community outreach, assistance in finding supportive living arrangements, and/or assertive community treatment (see Appendix B), as well as exploration of systems incentives to consolidate engagement in treatment. (This is an important consideration because of the potential consequences of relapse or continued use, such as loss of employment, loss of child custody, incarceration due to violation of probation, development of serious liver disease, etc.). Utilization of any available external leverage and incentives is critical.

The patient also may need recovery support services, such as help with housing, employment, education, and the like.</td>
<td>Monitoring for and managing any transient side effects may require a medically monitored inpatient (Level III.7) level of care.

Setting and Service Delivery

Significant severity may reflect acuity and/or chronicity. Circumstances that reflect high acuity (without imminent danger, which would denote a Risk Rating of 4) tend to warrant high-intensity interventions, especially in patients who appear able to engage in and respond to the types of interventions typically found at Dimension 4. For example, such a placement may involve a Level III.3 or Level III.5 setting (or Level III.7 if Risk Rating 3 or 4 service needs have been identified in Dimensions 1, 2, or 3).

Alternatively, Level II services may be used for clinical therapies in combination with Level III.1 clinically managed low-intensity residential services.

Patients whose circumstances reflect high chronicity but lower acuity may respond better to lower intensity interventions and levels of care. In some circumstances, patients with high chronicity and low readiness to change (Dimension 4) are unlikely to benefit from services that otherwise might meet their needs because they are unable to engage in those services. In such situations, the goal should be to match the patient's significant severity with increased duration rather than more intensive services.

Other patients with high chronicity may benefit from more intensive interventions and higher levels of care if they are likely to be engaged in those services, or if lower intensity services have failed or are likely to fail, or if their service needs in Dimension 4 dictate the greater intensity.

Total treatment dose may be increased through use of strategies that increase engagement at a less intensive level of care over a longer period of time (sometimes including continuing care). For example, such a placement may involve a Level I or II outpatient addiction or psychiatric program (a "dual diagnosis capable" or "dual diagnosis enhanced" service, depending on the level of severity in Dimension 3), with assertive case management or assertive community treatment and a supportive living arrangement.</td>
</tr>
</table>

(continues)

RISK RATING	SERVICE NEEDS AND INTERVENTIONS	LEVEL OF CARE AND SETTING
cravings to use, but he or she is *not* at risk of imminent harm. Or the patient's uninterrupted drinking may have led to chronic homelessness, which is chronically unsafe but not imminently dangerous (except where there *is* some acute danger such as the risk of exposure in freezing weather, in which case the Risk Rating would be **4**).		Initiation of medication therapy in the context of the high-intensity engagement supports typically found in residential treatment can help to reinforce medication adherence. The residential levels of care also can provide intensive role induction, which is helpful with pharmacologic therapies as well as other treatment interventions. Pharmacotherapy for alcohol dependence should be a standard component of the services provided by residential/inpatient treatment programs. Clinically monitored and clinically managed levels of care can provide such services through integrated or closely coordinated networks of providers. The medically monitored levels of care should have staff (such as physicians, physician extenders, and nurses) in place to evaluate patients and prescribe or administer antiaddiction medications as needed. At this intensity of treatment, addiction counselors should have a central role in supporting pharmacotherapies, particularly with regard to medication adherence and monitoring the patient's response to treatment. Programs should have mechanisms in place (such as training, supervision, and documentation) to foster and support such activities. In planning for ongoing care that will follow intensive treatment at this level of care, special attention should be given to the need for ongoing patient monitoring and medication management. This can be performed by an appropriately experienced primary care physician or a specialist in addiction medicine or addiction psychiatry.
Risk Rating = 4 (Severe risk) A Risk Rating of **4** indicates that the patient's acute condition places him or her at *severe risk* for relapse to or continuation of substance use. Such a patient lacks the skills to arrest his or her	**Service Needs** ***(Note: Immediate action is required.)*** A Risk Rating of **4** indicates imminent danger and an urgent need for specific professional services to address the patient's severe risk of relapse or continued use in Dimension 5. The patient with a Risk Rating of **4** needs containment for stabilization while imminently dangerous. Such a patient may appear committed to continued alcohol use, which his or her history indicates will lead to suicidal or homicidal behavior, dangerous impulses, or problems with self-care.	**Level of Care** The patient with a Risk Rating of **4** requires containment for stabilization while he or she is imminently dangerous. A Risk Rating of **4** usually indicates the need for Level IV medically managed intensive inpatient services, where the patient can receive medical or psychiatric close observation for his or her dangerous, impulsive behavior. Alternatively, Level III.7 medically monitored services may be appropriate if the intensity of medical or psychiatric close observation and management is sufficient.

substance use (*see the guide to the determination of risk ratings*).

The severity of the patient's risk of relapse or continued use indicates that he or she may pose an imminent danger to self and others. For example, the patient's continued substance use may lead to suicidal, psychotic, or aggressive behaviors; dangerous medical consequences (such as gastrointestinal bleeding or acute pancreatitis); or dangerously impulsive behaviors (such as repeatedly driving while intoxicated).

Such a patient typically has an extensive history of use, marked by high levels of severity and possibly chronicity, with the important qualifier that the current episode is characterized by high acuity, with imminently dangerous consequences.

Severity in other dimensions also may interact with risk in Dimension 5 in such a way that the patient requires containment and stabilization. For example, if a patient is physically dependent and at risk for severe withdrawal, supervised detoxification/managed withdrawal in a residential or inpatient setting is very strongly recommended (*refer to Dimension 1*).

If the patient is (or is likely to become) suicidal or homicidal or to have self-care problems (Dimension 3), containment with appropriate psychiatric treatment is very strongly recommended.

If the patient is at imminent risk of dangerous medical consequences (Dimension 2), containment with appropriate medical treatment is very strongly recommended.

Treatment Interventions

High-intensity relapse prevention services are urgently needed (*see the discussions in Chapters 4 and 5, as well as Appendix B particularly the list of core interventions in Table 6-3*). At this level of severity, patients need very aggressive management and should be offered the full range of available treatments.

Patients with a Risk Rating of **4** typically have failed previous interventions and should be offered new treatment modalities and adjunctive therapies as part of a comprehensive treatment plan.

In the absence of contraindications, initiation of treatment with an antiaddiction medication should be very strongly considered. Pharmacotherapies should be available as a routine component of treatment for patients with a Risk Rating of **4**.

The patient with a Risk Rating of **4** typically needs help with compliance/adherence to the various components of the treatment plan, including pharmacotherapies. Utilization of any available external leverage and incentives is crucial.

If the patient's degree of impulsivity requires 24-hour structure but not medical or psychiatric close observation, Level III.5 clinically managed residential services may be appropriate.

The patient who has co-occurring substance use and medical or psychiatric disorders may require more intensive services than would a patient with one disorder alone. If a Level III.7 or Level IV Dual Diagnosis Enhanced service is indicated but not available, the patient should be placed in an inpatient psychiatric service and stabilized before being referred for addiction treatment.

The need to monitor for and manage any transient side effects may be an added indication for a medically monitored inpatient level of care (Level III.7). In some situations, residential/inpatient monitoring may be necessary to establish the lead-in period of abstinence recommended before therapy with an antiaddiction medication is initiated. The residential and inpatient levels of care also can provide intensive role induction, which is helpful for pharmacologic therapies as well as for other treatment interventions.

Initiation of medications in the context of the high intensity supports typically found in medically monitored or managed treatment can help reinforce medication adherence.

Setting and Service Delivery

Pharmacotherapy for alcohol dependence should be a standard component of the services offered by residential/inpatient programs.

Medically monitored and medically managed levels of care should have staff (such as physicians, physician-extenders, and nurses) in place to evaluate patients and prescribe or administer antiaddiction medications.

Once the patient has been stabilized, a step down to a high-intensity but less restrictive continuing care setting usually is indicated. A supervised supportive living arrangement should be strongly considered (*refer to Dimension 6*).

In planning for the period of less intensive, longer term care that will follow treatment at this level of care, special attention should be given to the need for ongoing monitoring and medication management. This can be performed by an appropriately experienced primary care physician or a specialist in addiction medicine or addiction psychiatry.

CHAPTER 7

Case Examples of Risk Assessment

INTRODUCTION

The following case presentations are designed to illustrate how a clinician would go about assessing risk in each of the six ASAM Dimensions in order to create a severity profile, both at the time of initial assessment and at periodic reassessment. The cases also illustrate the effect on the overall risk rating of interactions among the various Dimensions (see the discussion of Dimensional Interaction, Table 2-1, pages 15–22).

In addition to presenting a conceptual organization for assessing risk in all six ASAM Dimensions, the cases give particular attention to Dimension 5, using the constructs and criteria developed for the ASAM *Patient Placement Criteria Supplement on Pharmacotherapy for Alcohol Use Disorders,* as well as the full criteria in PPC-2R. Several of the Cases (Cases 2 and 7) also give additional attention to Dimension 1. These assessment examples employ the four domains described in Chapter 6 (see pages 99–101) and offer a conceptually clear sequence of factors to be used in patient assessment.

CASE 1: MRS. A

Abstract

This case illustrates:

- Rational treatment planning, following a sequence that moves from assessment to specific treatment service needs, and finally to level of care.
- The role of recovery environment (Dimension 6) in determining the treatment plan and placement decisions.
- Strategies for managing severe relapse risk in a high-intensity outpatient level of care.
- Considerations in deciding whether to add pharmacotherapy to a multimodality treatment regimen.

Initial Presentation

Mrs. A, a 32-year-old woman, has been referred for assessment by her primary care physician. She has been diagnosed with alcohol dependence, marijuana abuse, and major depressive disorder.

She has been abstinent from alcohol for 72 hours and reports that she has maintained sobriety for up to 3 days during the preceding 3 months. She reports that, during these periods of abstinence, she has experienced sweating, tremors, and nausea, but has never had hallucinations, delirium tremens, or seizures.

Mrs. A is in good health except for acute alcoholic hepatitis, for which she was released from the hospital 1 week earlier. She had mild withdrawal symptoms on admission to the hospital and resumed drinking following discharge. However, she has not had withdrawal symptoms since stopping drinking 3 days ago. She smokes up to two or three marijuana cigarettes a day, but stopped yesterday.

Mrs. A describes two past suicide attempts using sleeping pills. The most recent attempt was 3 years ago. She sees a psychiatrist once a month for treatment of depression, and takes a selective serotonin reuptake inhibitor (SSRI) (fluoxetine/Prozac®) at the prescribed dose and frequency. Her mood is anxious and low, but she is not hopeless or suicidal.

Mrs. A, who is divorced, lives in an apartment with her 11-year-old son (who, she says, does not complain about her drinking and is unaware of her marijuana use). She has few friends since moving to a new area following her divorce a year ago. She is unemployed, having lost her job when the department store where she worked closed. In the past, she worked as a waitress, checkout clerk, and retail salesperson and says she has never lost a job because of drinking.

Mrs. A speaks calmly and is cooperative. She is not sweating, nauseated, or tremulous. She says she wants help. She shows awareness of the consequences of her substance use, but tends to minimize them and to blame others, including her ex-husband, who left her without warning. She appears to have little understanding of alcoholism or drug addiction, but wants to know more.

Dimensional Assessment

Dimension 1 (Acute Intoxication/Withdrawal Potential) Mrs. A has not had a drink for 72 hours and shows no evidence of withdrawal (e.g., she is "calm and cooperative"). Given her history of no more than moderate withdrawal symptoms (and even considering her use of marijuana, which might have minimal effects on reducing withdrawal symptoms, e.g., minimal effects on anxiety, some antiemetic effect), her risk of acute withdrawal has apparently passed, resulting in a Risk Rating of 0 (*minimal or no observable risk*). The effect of the fluoxetine on withdrawal must be considered (none), as well as the effect of possible liver dysfunction secondary to the alcoholic hepatitis (given 3 days of abstinence and no current withdrawal symptoms, this is not currently an issue). Therefore, no detoxification services are indicated.

Dimension 2 (Biomedical Conditions and Complications) The fact that Mrs. A was discharged from the hospital suggests that her problems in Dimension 2 are stabilizing. The appropriate treatment intervention for her hepatitis is abstinence from alcohol and any other hepatotoxic substance. However, she resumed drinking between 1 and 5 days postdischarge, and the effect on her liver function is not known. Her primary care physician should be consulted for a current assessment of liver function. Pending receipt of that information, the most appropriate Risk Rating is 2 (*moderate risk*).

Dimension 3 (Emotional/Behavioral/Cognitive Conditions and Complications) Mrs. A's history of suicide attempts and depression are of concern. However, the most recent suicide attempt was 3 years ago and a very stressful intervening event (her husband leaving her without warning) did not exacerbate her condition to the point of suicidality. Mrs. A is being treated for depression and is following the prescribed treatment regimen except for the recommendation not to drink. Based on this information alone, her Risk Rating would be 1 (*mild risk*) in Dimension 3. However, Mrs. A's status in other dimensions also must be considered. For example, her current status (and presumed stability) occurs in the context of her use of a combination of fluoxetine, cannabis, and alcohol, and it is unclear what effect a change in this complex psychoactive formula would have. Additionally, she has many stressors in Dimension 6 (she is an unemployed single parent who lacks a social support system), and these have the potential to increase her risk in Dimension 3. Thus, her overall Risk Rating in Dimension 3 would be 2 (*moderate risk*). While Mrs. A does not appear to need additional mental health services at this time, it would be advantageous to monitor her level of depression once she is fully withdrawn from alcohol (and possibly cannabis) and engaged in recovery services.

Dimension 4 (Readiness to Change) Mrs. A's status in this Dimension is characterized by ambivalence (e.g., "Mrs. A shows awareness of the consequences of her alcohol and drug use, but tends to minimize them and/or to blame others, including her ex-husband" and "She appears to have little understanding of alcoholism or drug addiction, but wants to know more"). Mrs. A kept the appointment for assessment, is cooperative, and says she wants to learn more about alcoholism, suggesting that she is in at least the *Contemplation* stage of change. The appropriate Risk Rating is 1 (*mild risk*). However, she will need active education and engagement strategies to sustain her initial willingness and to help her progress through the readiness to change continuum.

Dimension 5 (Relapse/Continued Use/Continued Problem Potential) Mrs. A's history and pattern of use are substantial, based on her history and pattern of substance use: her inability to remain abstinent from alcohol for more than 72 hours, her concurrent use of marijuana, and the fact that she resumed alcohol use within 1 day of being discharged from the hospital after being treated for alcoholic hepatitis. We do not know enough about her response to substance effects or cognitive and behavioral measures of temperament, vulnerabilities, and resilience. The stressors that exist in Dimension 6 (Mrs. A is an unemployed, single parent who lacks a social support system) further increase her risk in Dimension 5, although this is mediated to some extent by her readiness to change (Dimension 4).

Overall, Mrs. A appears to be at very high risk for continued alcohol and drug use, resulting in a Risk Rating of 3 (*significant risk*). If we were to learn that the severity of her liver problem or other features of her medical condition placed her in imminent danger, then we would change this to 4 (*severe risk, with imminent danger*).

Dimension 6 (Recovery Environment) As noted previously, Mrs. A has many stressors in this Dimension, but she does have a place to live that is not actively toxic. She also has job skills that could allow reemployment and she does have custody of her son, about whom she is concerned. However, her belief that her son is unaffected by her drinking and unaware of her marijuana use appears to be at odds with what would be expected and a session with her son to gather further information is in order. Mrs. A will need vocational help and perhaps temporary financial assistance until she is working again. In this Dimension, her Risk Rating is 3 (*significant risk*).

Placement and Discussion

Dimension 5 is the area in which Mrs. A is assessed as having the greatest severity and vulnerability, so the treatment plan should focus on strategies and supports to help Mrs. A maintain abstinence in the near term, given her history of maintaining sobriety for no more than 72 hours, particularly significant since Mrs. A is now at the 72-hour point and her history would predict that she would return to drinking without active intervention. Thus, maintaining abstinence for more than 72 hours can provide a short-term treatment goal and achieving it can be reinforcing (and should be praised) as an early treatment success. Mrs. A's immediate service needs are for close support, especially over the next 24 hours, as she deals with cravings and impulses to resume use. A session with her son also is very important to assure that he is safe and not subject to neglect.

Mrs. A could be placed in a day treatment program (Level II.5), at least for a few days, to ensure that her potential for continued use is sufficiently under control. If she appears unable to resist cravings to use, additional supports will be necessary. For example, she may be willing and able to use the support of frequent self-help recovery group meetings in conjunction with volunteers from those groups providing companionship over the next 24 to 48 hours. As an alternative, the support of a relative or friend might be recruited. If Mrs. A becomes successfully integrated into a self-help recovery group, then subsequent continued service in an intensive outpatient (Level II.1) program may be safe and appropriate. However, if she still manifests considerable ambivalence, then continued service in a Level II.5 program is indicated for safety reasons.

Given her current issues in Dimension 3, placement in a Dual Diagnosis Capable program should be considered. If this is not available at Level II.5, then consideration should be given to placing Mrs. A in a clinically managed low-intensity residential (Level III.1) program that treats women and children (although some of these programs will not accept a child the age of Mrs. A's son), in combination with Level II.5 addiction treatment program. Because Mrs. A does not pose an imminent danger to self or others, other residential or inpatient placements would be clinically inappropriate.

Given her history and pattern of use, strong consideration should be given to prescribing an antiaddiction medication for Mrs. A. Given her recent history of hepatitis, Mrs. A's liver function tests should be monitored closely to confirm her progress (naltrexone and disulfiram should be avoided if her liver function remains severely impaired, although both are less hepatotoxic than alcohol). If the Level II.5 program in which she is placed is not affiliated with a physician, others who might prescribe an antiaddiction medication include her psychiatrist or her primary care physician with close collaboration with the addiction treatment program. Use of antiaddiction medications should be followed through frequent medication management sessions to

TABLE 7-1A

Mrs. A's Initial Dimensional Severity Profile

	Risk Rating				
ASAM Dimension	*0 Minimal or no observable risk*	*1 Mild risk*	*2 Moderate risk*	*3 Significant risk*	*4 Severe risk*
Dimension 1: Acute Intoxication and/or Withdrawal Potential	X				
Dimension 2: Biomedical Conditions and Complications			X*		
Dimension 3: Emotional, Behavioral, and Cognitive Conditions and Complications			X		
Dimension 4: Readiness to Change		X			
Dimension 5: Relapse/Continued Use/Continued Problem Potential				X	
Dimension 6: Recovery Environment				X	

* More information is needed about Mrs. A's liver function, which may lead to a change in this Risk Rating.

reinforce adherence, assess response, and monitor progress. The intensive support of a Level II.5 program presents a valuable opportunity to achieve some of these goals and to integrate pharmacotherapy with psychosocial interventions. It is critical that the program staff understand, support, and reinforce the goals of the pharmacotherapy. Cross-training should help counselors monitor medication adherence, medication side effects, and medication response.

In cases such as that of Mrs. A, gaps in the continuum of care may be exposed. Such gaps often lead to placements at the most intensive levels of care (such as Level III.5, Clinically Managed High Intensity Residential Treatment, or Level III.7, Medically Monitored Intensive Inpatient Treatment) as a way to assure that the patient's needs are being met. However, use of higher than necessary levels of care (assuming that others are available) is not appropriate clinically, deploys resources inefficiently, and impedes access to those who do need those levels of intensity.

Other issues that need to be considered are the absence of a positive social support system for Mrs. A, which can be addressed through involvement in a self-help recovery group. Also, a review of Mrs. A's employment history does not indicate specific job skills but does highlight an apparent strength in her ability to interact with the public. Vocational assessment and possible vocational training for a set of specific job skills should be considered.

Another issue to be addressed is Mrs. A's use of marijuana. Ideally, Mrs. A would have as a goal abstinence from both alcohol and marijuana, particularly because continued marijuana use could increase the likelihood of continued alcohol use. However, if Mrs. A is unable to stop her use of marijuana at this time, initial focus should be placed on cessation of alcohol use because of her alcoholic hepatitis, accompanied by motivational enhancement strategies to support her abstinence from marijuana.

Findings at Follow-up: Reassessment

At a follow-up visit 4 months later, Mrs. A reports that she has been abstinent from alcohol for almost 4 months. She has transitioned well to less intensive levels of outpatient care, has been discharged from a Level I program, and is attending self-help group meetings two to three times a week. She has not used marijuana for the past 2 weeks. Her liver function test results are within normal limits.

However, Mrs. A discloses that her sister, from whom she had been estranged, died recently, before they could reestablish their relationship. Mrs. A feels guilt that she was unable to bring about a rapprochement. She also has become involved in a relationship that she describes as being "madly in love." The man in question moved in with her, but shortly thereafter she discovered him being sexually unfaithful. She has fallen into a deep depression even though she continues to use her antidepressant medication.

Mrs. A reports that, for the first time in 3 years, she occasionally thinks about suicide, although she says she does not have an active plan and is willing to make a safety contract. She reports that she is barely able to care for her son. Mrs. A started a new job as a salesperson, but is still in her initial probationary period and has called in sick for the past 3 days.

Dimension 1 (Acute Intoxication/Withdrawal Potential) Mrs. A continues to be stable, with no observable problem, resulting in a Risk Rating of 0 (*minimal or no observable risk*).

Dimension 2 (Biomedical Conditions and Complications) Mrs. A's improved liver function supports a downgrading of her Risk Rating to 0 (*minimal or no observable risk*).

Dimension 3 (Emotional/Behavioral/Cognitive Conditions and Complications) Mrs. A's risk in this Dimension has sharply increased because of the return of her depression and suicidal ideation, both of which render her history of suicide attempts more of a concern. While some of her stressors in Dimension 6 have resolved (e.g., she is now employed), others are still present and new one have developed (e.g., problems in her new relationship). Therefore, her Risk Rating has increased to 3 (*significant risk*). (If there was greater concern about Mrs. A's suicidality, a Risk Rating of 3 might be warranted. If she was assessed as imminently dangerous (e.g., unable to make a credible safety contract), her Risk Rating would be 4.

Dimension 4 (Readiness to Change) Mrs. A appears to be in the Action stage in terms of her treatment engagement and motivation to stop her substance use. Therefore, in Dimension 4, her Risk Rating is 0 (*minimal or no observable risk*).

Dimension 5 (Relapse/Continued Use/Continued Problem Potential) Mrs. A's risk in Dimension 5 ordinarily would be considered minimal. Her recent pattern of alcohol and marijuana use is not severe, she has had a positive response to intervention, and there is no indication of significant risk in terms of her response to substance effects. However, the recurrence of Mrs. A's

TABLE 7-1B

Mrs. A's Dimensional Severity Profile at Follow-up

	Risk Rating				
ASAM Dimension	*0 Minimal or no observable risk*	*1 Mild risk*	*2 Moderate risk*	*3 Significant risk*	*4 Severe risk*
Dimension 1: Acute Intoxication and/or Withdrawal Potential	X				
Dimension 2: Biomedical Conditions and Complications	X				
Dimension 3: Emotional, Behavioral, and Cognitive Conditions and Complications				X	
Dimension 4: Readiness to Change	X				
Dimension 5: Relapse/Continued Use/Continued Problem Potential				X	
Dimension 6: Recovery Environment				X	

depressive symptoms and suicidal ideation indicate that she is at substantial risk for continued problems. It can be assumed that stressors in Dimension 6 may be contributing to her risk level. Given these factors, she is assigned a Risk Rating of 3 (*significant risk*) in Dimension 5.

Dimension 6 (Recovery Environment) Mrs. A's stressors either still exist (e.g., she is a single mother) or they have been replaced by other stressors (e.g., her unemployment has been replaced by a level of job performance that may cost her employment). Her reported difficulty in caring for her son may possibly put her son at risk. Her severity in this Dimension is considered significant, for a Risk Rating of 3.

Placement and Discussion

Mrs. A's actions that support continued sobriety (such as her participation in self-help recovery groups) should be reinforced and an increase in frequency should be suggested. Mrs. A does not need to be readmitted to an addiction treatment program, but her psychiatric treatment should be intensified. She should be reevaluated by her psychiatrist, with follow-up at more frequent intervals. Counseling and/or psychotherapy should address her relationship with her sister and the grief she feels, her feelings of betrayal by her romantic partner and her judgment about that relationship, and coaching about her job functioning. It is especially important that such counseling include explicit discussion and monitoring of her heightened relapse risk. Consideration also should be given to adjusting her antidepressant medication.

Mrs. A's suicide risk should be monitored frequently and, if she becomes actively suicidal, her placement should be stepped up to a more intensive level of care. If she experiences a relapse to alcohol use, she should be readmitted immediately to addiction treatment, and her suicide risk would increase substantially, possibly placing her in imminent danger. If she is not already taking an antiaddiction medication, strong consideration should be given to adding one to her treatment regimen, at least during the period of instability.

Summary

This case illustrates rational treatment planning, following a sequence that moves first from assessment to specific treatment service needs and finally to level of care. It features strategies for managing severe relapse risk in a high-intensity outpatient level of care, and explores the rationale for adding pharmacotherapy to a multimodality treatment regimen. It also highlights the need for ongoing monitoring and the possible need for other treatment after the conclusion of the formal addiction treatment.

CASE 2: MR. B

Abstract

This case illustrates:

- Rational treatment planning with a patient who is at very high risk for withdrawal.
- The contribution of both history and pattern of substance use, as well as response to substance effects, in assessing relapse risk (Dimension 5).

- Considerations in deciding whether to add pharmacotherapy to a multimodality treatment regimen.
- The role of mental health (Dimension 3) in mediating relapse risk (Dimension 5). This is an important example of interdimensional risk.
- The role of recovery environment (Dimension 6) in determining the treatment plan and placement decisions.
- An example of treatment planning and placement in a case of very high Dimension 1 withdrawal risk

Initial Presentation

Mr. B, a 43-year-old man, has been referred for assessment after being cited for a DUI offense, at which time his blood alcohol level was 0.05 mg%. This was his second DUI citation within 5 weeks. His urine drug screen also was positive for marijuana, which he says he began to use about 30 days ago.

Mr. B, reports that he was admitted to a 28-day inpatient alcohol rehabilitation program 7 years ago. Following his discharge, he remained abstinent from alcohol for 18 months. He describes his current daily consumption as 8 to 10 bottles of beer on weekdays and 15 to 20 bottles a day on weekends. He last had a drink almost 18 hours before the assessment, and he is clearly agitated and grossly tremulous. His CIWA-Ar score is 22.

He has been divorced for 4 years and admits that his alcohol use contributed to the divorce. He does not currently have a significant other nor does he date much. Although he currently has custody of, and lives with, his two daughters, who are 16 and 13, his ex-wife has initiated a suit for custody.

Mr. B is employed as a technician by a heating and air conditioning company, with which he has 19 years of service. However, within the past 2 months, he has developed a pattern of tardiness and coworkers have noted the odor of alcohol on more than one occasion. Work-related stressors include a new position with the company and a possible temporary transfer (for 6 months) to a work site 160 miles away.

Mr. B recently was diagnosed with pancreatitis. He is experiencing mild pain, but is managing to eat a normal diet. He admits to feeling stressed and somewhat depressed, and to having fleeting suicidal ideation. He says he uses alcohol to alleviate his depression and loneliness. He has not been abstinent from alcohol for more than 2 days at a time within the past 5 years. When he does stop drinking, Mr. B says he experiences moderate to severe shakes and "passes out" (tentative diagnosis: withdrawal seizure). He has not attempted to stop drinking and describes his social support system as "weak." While Mr. B does not admit to being alcoholic, he is willing to enter treatment to keep his job.

Dimensional Assessment

Dimension 1 (Acute Intoxication/Withdrawal Potential) Given his pattern of drinking (especially his inability to abstain from alcohol for more than 2 consecutive days over the past 5 years), his probable withdrawal seizures, and his CIWA-Ar score of 22, Mr. B's risk in Dimension 1 is assessed as severe, for a Risk Rating of 4 (*severe risk*).

Dimension 2 (Biomedical Conditions and Complications) Although Mr. B has only mild symptoms at present, the instability of active pancreatitis justifies a Risk Rating of 2 (*moderate risk*).

Dimension 3 (Emotional/Behavioral/Cognitive Conditions and Complications) Mr. B describes himself as feeling stressed, somewhat depressed, and with fleeting suicidal ideation. These factors suggest a Risk Rating of 2 (*moderate risk*) in this Dimension.

Dimension 4 (Readiness to Change) The patient appears to be motivated to do whatever is needed to keep his job and could be described as in an Action stage of change regarding his work. However, he does not believe he is alcoholic, and is in the Precontemplation stage of change regarding his drinking. Therefore, his Risk Rating in Dimension 4 is 3 (*significant risk*).

Dimension 5 (Relapse/Continued Use/Continued Problem Potential) Mr. B evidences a chronic pattern of use (e.g., no more than 2 consecutive days' abstinence in the past 5 years) and considerable severity (consumption of 8 to 20 bottles of beer per day). Although he had an excellent response to treatment 7 years ago, more recently he has shown a very poor response to change (i.e., to a diagnosis of pancreatitis and two DUIs within a 5-week period). These recent sequelae also indicate a severe level of risk.

It appears that Mr. B is at moderate risk in terms of his response to substance effects (with likely negative reinforcement of drinking, that is the alleviation of negative effects of abstinence, e.g., use of alcohol to relieve his feelings of being stressed, depressed, and suicidal, as well as his use of alcohol to alleviate symptoms of withdrawal).

We have no information about his response to external stimuli such as stress cues and triggers. With regard to cognitive and behavioral measures of temperament, vulnerabilities, and resilience, Mr. B appears to have difficulty in coping and dealing effectively with challenges and adversity (of which he currently has a considerable number). It appears that stressors in Dimension 6 are contributing to his continued use. Even though his past treatment and ensuing 18 months of abstinence mediate Mr. B's risk level to some extent, a Risk Rating of 3 (*significant risk*) is justified by his current level of function. If his pancreatitis symptoms again became more severe and debilitating, this would indicate imminent danger and an increase in Risk Rating to 4 (severe risk).

Dimension 6 (Recovery Environment) Mr. B's stressors include a new position in the company where he has been employed for 19 years, the prospect of a 6-month transfer to a company site 160 miles away, being a single working parent, and engaging in a custody suit initiated by his ex-wife. Therefore, his severity in this Dimension justifies a Risk Rating of 3 (*significant risk*).

Placement and Discussion

In prioritizing Mr. B's problems, it is clear that the first placement must be for management of withdrawal in a Level III.7-D, medically monitored inpatient detoxification service. During and after the withdrawal, Mr. B's Dimensions 3 issues of stress, depression, and suicidal ideation must be closely monitored.

The next most severe problem is the likelihood that Mr. B will continue his alcohol and marijuana use. Consideration should be given to intervention in his Dimension 6 issues (as by determining whether he has legal counsel to represent him in the custody suit, whether the company is willing to forego or delay his job transfer, etc.).

After Mr. B achieves several days of abstinence, initiation of an antiaddiction medication is strongly indicated. The medically monitored level of care is an excellent setting for the kind of role induction that is so helpful with pharmacologic therapies, as well as for initiating nonpharmacologic treatment services. Initiating the medication in the context of the high-intensity supports typically found in a Level III.7 program can help considerably in reinforcing medication adherence and helping the patient get through any transient side effects.

At Discharge From Detoxification: Reassessment

The patient has successfully completed detoxification. Although Mr. B no longer evidences physiologic signs of withdrawal, he has persistent insomnia and significant anxiety. He says that he really wants to stop drinking but is concerned that he will be unable to do so. His perception of the best option for him, based on his experience 7 years ago, is treatment in a residential program similar to the 28-day inpatient rehabilitation center where he was treated last time. However, he does not know how to reconcile that with his child care obligations or the upcoming job transfer.

TABLE 7-2A

Mr. B's Initial Dimensional Severity Profile

	Risk Rating				
ASAM Dimension	*0 Minimal or no observable risk*	*1 Mild risk*	*2 Moderate risk*	*3 Significant risk*	*4 Severe risk*
Dimension 1: Acute Intoxication and/or Withdrawal Potential					X
Dimension 2: Biomedical Conditions and Complications			X		
Dimension 3: Emotional, Behavioral, and Cognitive Conditions and Complications			X		
Dimension 4: Readiness to Change				X	
Dimension 5: Relapse/Continued Use/Continued Problem Potential				X	
Dimension 6: Recovery Environment				X	

If anything, his anxiety, depression, and craving for alcohol have increased since he stopped drinking. He feels overwhelmed and intermittently hopeless, but is not suicidal.

Dimension 1 (Acute Intoxication/Withdrawal Potential) Acute withdrawal has responded to treatment though he continues to have lingering milder symptoms. In this Dimension his Risk Rating has decreased from 4 (*severe risk*) to 1 (*mild risk*).

Dimension 2 (Biomedical Conditions and Complications) Continued abdominal pain and signs of pancreatic inflammation result in a continued Risk Rating of 2 (*moderate risk*).

Dimension 3 (Emotional/Behavioral/Cognitive Conditions and Complications) In this Dimension, Mr. B's Risk Rating has increased from 2 (*moderate risk*) to 3 (*significant risk*) because of his increased anxiety, depression, and feelings of being overwhelmed and hopeless.

Dimension 4 It appears that his readiness to change has shifted somewhat from wanting to stop drinking only to keep his job (external) to wanting to stop drinking for himself (internal). His concern that he will be unable to stop drinking is appropriate, given his history. Risk Rating has decreased from 3 to 2.

Dimension 5 (Relapse/Continued Use/Continued Problem Potential) Mr. B's risk of relapse remains at 3 (*significant risk*), as demonstrated by his recent history of substance use and the severity of his response to substance effects (i.e., his severe subjective cravings; his subjective sense of loss of control in relation to relief of feelings of being stressed, anxious, and depressed; and his expectation that alcohol would alleviate the persistent abstinence symptoms).

Placement and Discussion

Once Mr. B's detoxification is complete, the primary concerns become (1) his increased anxiety and depression, (2) his increased craving for alcohol, and (3) the possibility the he will relapse to drinking. On the positive side, it appears that his readiness to change and treatment engagement has improved. His concern that he will be unable to stop drinking is appropriate, given his history.

These issues support placement in a Dual Diagnosis Enhanced Level II.5 program, coupled with involvement in a recovery support group to address his weak social support system and issues in Dimension 3. Consideration could be given to placement in a Dual Diagnosis Enhanced Level III.5 program, but that would require special arrangements for the care of his daughters. (There is no information about a third party who could care for Mr. B's children.)

The other consideration that argues against such a placement is Mr. B's upcoming custody suit. He should be helped to understand that he has the ability to reachieve his previous treatment response and period of abstinence, and that he can do so without being admitted to a residential or inpatient program. Of course, if an appropriate II.5 program is not available, then other placements would need to be considered, including a residential program with suitable arrangements for the children.

He should be assessed for depression and possibly the need for antidepressant medication and counseling to address his stress, anxiety, and depression. In view of his medical problem, he also needs linkage to ongoing care.

TABLE 7-2B

Mr. B's Postdetoxification Dimensional Severity Profile

	Risk Rating				
ASAM Dimension	*0 Stable (no observable risk)*	*1 Mild Risk*	*2 Moderate Risk*	*3 Significant Risk*	*4 Severe Risk*
Dimension 1: Acute Intoxication and/or Withdrawal Potential		X			
Dimension 2: Biomedical Conditions and Complications			X		
Dimension 3: Emotional, Behavioral, and Cognitive Conditions and Complications				X	
Dimension 4: Readiness to Change			X		
Dimension 5: Relapse/Continued Use/Continued Problem Potential				X	
Dimension 6: Recovery Environment				X	

Mr. B continues to be a good candidate for an antiaddiction medication (acamprosate, oral naltrexone, or extended-release injectable naltrexone or disulfiram) because of his craving and relapse risk. This must be accompanied by ongoing medication management with frequent initial monitoring, either by an addiction medicine specialist, a primary care physician with addiction experience, or a less experienced prescriber in concert with an addiction clinician who has developed sophistication in supporting antiaddiction medication treatment.

Summary

This case illustrates rational treatment planning with a patient who is at very high risk for withdrawal.

CASE 3: MR. C

Abstract

This case illustrates:

- The contribution to relapse risk of factors such as cognitive and behavioral measures of temperament, vulnerability, and resiliency (Dimension 5).
- Considerations in deciding whether to add pharmacotherapy to a multimodality treatment regimen.
- The need to attend to recovery environment (Dimension 6) as a major factor in treatment planning and placement decisions.
- The importance of utilizing recovery support interventions that are not typically considered "treatment" as part of a treatment plan.
- An example of treatment planning requiring adaptation to the local array of resources, in which not all levels of care are available, including the notion of "weaving" together resources from locally available levels of care that can approximate one that is unavailable

Initial Presentation

Mr. C, a 66-year-old man, has come to the attention of an employee assistance program (EAP) counselor through a telephone call from his adult daughter, who lives out of state. While visiting her father, she found him semi-intoxicated throughout the evening hours.

A widower who lives alone, Mr. C was given early retirement at age 63 by his long-time employer, a supermarket chain. At that time, his family and employer were not aware of any alcohol problem, although his friends knew him to be a daily drinker. He lives in a very small town. He no longer drives.

The EAP counselor arranged for Mr. C to be assessed by a physician with whom the company had a contract. On examination, the physician saw no evidence of withdrawal other than insomnia. Historically he has had no more than mild withdrawal symptoms.

Mr. C takes no medications with central nervous system (CNS) effects. He is a heavy smoker (two or more packs of cigarettes per day) with some evidence of chronic obstructive pulmonary disease. Also, his liver is enlarged on physical examination, and his liver function tests are moderately elevated (2–3 times normal). There are no other medical problems of significance.

When asked about his alcohol use, Mr. C says that he "drinks practically every day," has done so for 20 years, and wants help to stop. He says that he can reduce his drinking to one or two times a week "if I really try." On several occasions, he has been able to abstain from alcohol for as long as a week

The patient has been mildly depressed since the death of his wife 2 years ago. He feels lonely much of the time and, when drinking, thinks about "ending it all," but his suicidal ideation has never progressed to the planning stage. He says his brief periods of sobriety ended when he began to think about the loss of his wife. Then he became pessimistic that he could manage on his own, or even that there was any point in stopping because he is alone. Being at home alone exacerbates his sense of loneliness, estrangement from others, and grief over the loss of his spouse.

Dimensional Assessment

Dimension 1 (Acute Intoxication/Withdrawal Potential) Given his CIWA-Ar score of 7 and his history of no more than mild withdrawal problems, Mr. C's Risk Rating in this Dimension is 0 (*minimal or no observable risk*). No detoxification services are indicated, other than perhaps a mild non–habit-forming sleep aid (such as low-dose trazodone or diphenhydramine) for insomnia.

Dimension 2 (Biomedical Conditions and Complications) Mr. C has two problems in Dimension 2: chronic obstructive pulmonary disease (COPD) and hepatic inflammation. Given that he is currently a heavy smoker, smoking cessation should be a goal to forestall the progression of his COPD. Abstinence from alcohol also should be a goal because of his hepatitis. His Risk Rating is 2 (*moderate risk*).

Dimension 3 (Emotional/Behavioral/Cognitive Conditions and Complications) The most striking issues in Dimension 3 are Mr. C's depression and unresolved grief over the death of his wife. Given his suicidal ideation (and particularly because men older than age 65 have a high rate of suicide), the patient should be assigned a Risk Rating of 2 (*moderate risk*).

Dimension 4 (Readiness to Change) Mr. C has intermittently tried to stop drinking, which suggests recognition that he has a problem. He thus appears to be somewhere between Contemplation and Preparation in the stages of change, but he does not have the skills or help to sustain his attempts at abstinence. Motivational enhancement therapy should also be initiated for smoking cessation, particularly in light of his COPD. In this Dimension, his Risk Rating is 1 (*mild risk*).

Dimension 5 (Relapse/Continued Use/Continued Problem Potential) Mr. C's pattern of use is of moderate severity, and he has demonstrated an ability to remain abstinent for up to a week at a time without outside help. It appears that there is moderate risk in terms of his response to substance effects (which appear to relieve his feelings of grief, depression, and loneliness). There is no indication of a significant response to external stimuli.

In regards to cognitive and behavioral measures of temperament, vulnerabilities, and resiliency, Mr. C appears to have difficulty in coping with the loss of his wife and he is pessimistic about his ability to change. Taken together, these findings support a Risk Rating of 2 (*moderate risk*) in this Dimension. There is a strong interdimensional contribution from Dimension 6 in terms of Mr. C's social situation and loneliness.

Dimension 6 (Recovery Environment) In this Dimension, Mr. C's major issue is his loneliness and estrangement from others. His severity in this Dimension is considered substantial, leading to a Risk Rating of 3 (*significant risk*).

Placement and Discussion

Mr. C's highest priority problem appears to be in Dimension 6, Recovery Environment, because of his loneliness and the apparent absence of a support system. He also has a moderately severe problem in Dimension 3, Emotional/Behavioral/Cognitive Conditions and Complications, because of unresolved grief over the death of his wife. To address this problem, Mr. C needs a psychiatric evaluation and may need psychiatric treatment concurrently with his addiction treatment. This could involve counseling focused on his grief, the use of antidepressant medication, suicide risk monitoring, and the like.

Mr. C also has problems in Dimension 2, Biomedical Conditions and Complications, as evidenced by his COPD and enlarged liver, but he is not in acute distress. Medical treatment for his COPD should include a smoking cessation program, either through the addiction treatment program or as an overlay to the program, possibly using pharmacotherapy (e.g., nicotine replacement therapy plus another smoking cessation medication, such as bupropion or varenicline) and smoking cessation counseling. His liver function should be monitored. Consideration should be given to the prescription of an antiaddiction medication to help him stop drinking (acamprosate, oral naltrexone, extended release injectable naltrexone, or disulfiram).

Based on his readiness to change (Dimension 4), Mr. C could be placed in a Level I (outpatient) program. However, his social isolation and lack of a support system argue for more structure and intensity, as is found in a Level II.1 intensive outpatient program. However, the nearest intensive outpatient program (IOP) is 65 miles away and Mr. C does not drive.

TABLE 7-3

Mr. C's Initial Dimensional Severity Profile

	Risk Rating				
ASAM Dimension	*0 Minimal or no observable risk*	*1 Mild risk*	*2 Moderate risk*	*3 Significant risk*	*4 Severe risk*
Dimension 1: Acute Intoxication and/or Withdrawal Potential	X				
Dimension 2: Biomedical Conditions and Complications			X		
Dimension 3: Emotional, Behavioral, and Cognitive Conditions and Complications			X		
Dimension 4: Readiness to Change		X			
Dimension 5: Relapse/Continued Use/Continued Problem Potential			X		
Dimension 6: Recovery Environment				X	

Three approaches might be used to resolve this placement dilemma:

1. A volunteer (such as an AA member) might be recruited to drive Mr. C to the IOP program, in exchange for reimbursement of expenses.
2. There may be an IOP program near where his daughter lives, and she may be willing to have her father live with her while he attends treatment.
3. A multidimensional program could be created by integrating a variety of services that approximate the intensity of an IOP program. For example, Mr. C could attend outpatient counseling sessions two to three times a week, attend a smoking cessation program, see a psychiatrist and/or primary care physician, attend a senior center daily for the structure and social support it provides, attend three AA meetings a week, and obtain an AA sponsor.

In addition, if Mr. C is treated with an antiaddiction medication as indicated, he will need ongoing medication management and frequent initial monitoring. This can be accomplished by his primary care physician. In that case, the addiction counselor(s) involved in his care will have to develop some skills in supporting antiaddiction medication therapy in close coordination with the prescriber.

Summary

This case illustrates that some important objectives of a treatment plan can be met by recovery support services such as transportation assistance that are not traditionally considered "treatment" (examples of other such services might include such as literacy training, vocational training, child care, and the like).

CASE 4: MRS. D

Abstract

This case illustrates:

- The role of history and pattern of substance use (Domain A), response to substance effects (Domain B), response to external stimuli (Domain C), and cognitive and behavioral measures of temperament, vulnerability, and resilience (Domain D) in assessing Dimension 5 relapse risk (see Chapter 6 for a description of these Domains).
- Considerations in deciding whether to add pharmacotherapy to a multimodality treatment regimen.

Initial Presentation

Mrs. D is a 45-year-old woman who was referred by a neighbor. She has been attending AA meetings off-and-on for about 2 years: "on" when she is sober and "off" when she is drinking. She claims to do well for periods of weeks to months, but then relapses. She reports that she initially imagines she can manage her drinking, but "just one" progresses to "just a few." Within a week or so, she has resumed her previous dependent level of consumption. Her pattern is to continue until she is interrupted by complaints from her family, problems at work, or other external pressures.

Mrs. D stopped drinking several days ago and has not experienced physiologic withdrawal symptoms. She says she is tired of not being able to control her drinking and wants help in maintaining her sobriety.

Initial Assessment

Dimension 1 (Acute Intoxication/Withdrawal Potential) Given the absence of a history of withdrawal problems, Mrs. D is assigned an initial Risk Rating of 0 (*minimal or no observable risk*). Therefore, no detoxification services are indicated.

Dimension 2 (Biomedical Conditions and Complications) There is no significant history of biomedical problems and no current or observable complaints, resulting in an initial Risk Rating of 0.

Dimension 3 (Emotional/Behavioral/Cognitive Conditions and Complications) There is no information to indicate a mental health problem, although Mrs. D has experienced recurrent difficulties with psychosocial functioning in terms of family life and work. This leads to an initial Risk Rating of 1 (*mild risk*), unless contradicted by further information.

Dimension 4 (Readiness to Change) Mrs. D appears to be in the Action Stage of Change, as evidenced by her attendance at AA meetings and her statement that she is unable to control her drinking and wants help. She seems to have preliminary motivation for abstinence. Thus, her initial Risk Rating is 1 (*mild risk*), but she needs further help with motivational enhancement.

Dimension 5 (Relapse/Continued Use/Continued Problem Potential) Mrs. D's pattern of use is of moderate severity, but significant chronicity. She has shown an inconsistent response to intervention (as demonstrated by 2 years' attendance at AA meetings without the ability to maintain abstinence). At the same time, Mrs. D exhibits a moderately positive response to external influences, and is intermittently able to stop drinking based on outside pressures (e.g., family, problems at work). At present, we have little information about her response to substance effects or to triggers or stressors. Similarly, there is little to indicate a significant response to external stimuli.

In terms of Mrs. D's cognitive and behavioral measures of temperament, vulnerabilities and resilience, current information suggests that she is having moderate difficulty in coping and dealing effectively with challenges and limitations. While she states that she has accepted her inability to control her drinking, there is some question as to the degree of her acceptance because she imagines she can manage her drinking, even though "just one" progresses to "just a few." She seems to be at least moderately passive in mobilizing personal resources to deal with risk or respond to resumption of dependence; for instance, she does not reach out for help until others pressure her to do so.

Taken together, Mrs. D's assessment in these domains leads to an initial Risk Rating of 2 (*moderate risk*).

Dimension 6 (Recovery Environment) The available information does not indicate a problem in this Dimension, leading to an initial Risk Rating of 0 (*minimal or no observable risk*).

TABLE 7-4A

Mrs. D's Initial Dimensional Severity Profile

	Risk Rating				
ASAM Dimension	*0 Minimal or no observable risk*	*1 Mild risk*	*2 Moderate risk*	*3 Significant risk*	*4 Severe risk*
Dimension 1: Acute Intoxication and/or Withdrawal Potential	X				
Dimension 2: Biomedical Conditions and Complications	X				
Dimension 3: Emotional, Behavioral, and Cognitive Conditions and Complications		X			
Dimension 4: Readiness to Change		X			
Dimension 5: Relapse/Continued Use/Continued Problem Potential			X		
Dimension 6: Recovery Environment	X				

Initial Placement

Based on the available information, it appears that the most appropriate placement for Mrs. D is a Level I outpatient program. Treatment should emphasize her inability to control her drinking and reinforce consistent AA involvement and the need to reach out for help when she initially lapses or more appropriately when she is even contemplating drinking. Consideration should be given to prescribing an antiaddiction medication to address her risk of relapse.

When the discussion of using an antiaddiction medication was raised, Mrs. D declined and made clear her opposition to the use of any antiaddiction medication. Further exploration of her resistance resulted in a decision not to pursue the medication option, even though it was the clinician's opinion that it was the best course. Mrs. D was encouraged to fully involve herself in AA on the grounds that, if it was successful, there would be no need to add antiaddiction medication.

Reassessment at Three Weeks (Scenario 1)

Mrs. D has been attending a Level I outpatient treatment program, and her work and family life are beginning to improve. However, she has lapsed over the past few days, admitting that she once again gave in to the temptation to have "just one or two." So far, she has used alcohol on three occasions, taking two drinks on two occasions and four drinks on another occasion. She reported that she has indeed increased her attendance at AA meetings but has not yet found a sponsor she is comfortable with.

As a result of her drinking episodes, she is less confident of her ability to control her drinking, but increasingly wonders again whether she might be able to manage it this time. On further discussion, she describes her lapses as often triggered by watching others enjoy drinking in social situations. She then thinks for several days about how good she would feel if she could have a drink. When she finally does take a drink, she enjoys it a great deal.

Dimension 1 (Acute Intoxication/Withdrawal Potential) There is no change in the initial Risk Rating of 0 (*minimal or no observable risk*).

Dimension 2 (Biomedical Conditions and Complications) There is no change in the initial Risk Rating of 0 (*minimal or no observable problems*).

Dimension 3 (Emotional/Behavioral/Cognitive Conditions and Complications) Mrs. D's improving psychosocial function indicates an adjusted Risk Rating of 1 (*mild risk*) or less.

Dimension 4 (Readiness to Change) Mrs. D remains motivated for treatment but is demonstrating increased ambivalence, as she begins to think that she might be able to control her drinking. This increases her Risk Rating to 2 (*moderate risk*).

Dimension 5 (Relapse/Continued Use/Continued Problem Potential) Mrs. D's lapses while in treatment raise concerns about the chronicity of her problem and her poor response to change. While her alcohol use is of moderate severity, she has been able to stop drinking in response to outside pressures (e.g., family, problems at work).

At this point, we have a better understanding of her response to substance effects; that is, Mrs. D derives significant reward and pleasure from drinking and her current pattern of use is providing significant positive reinforcement for continued and escalating use (reward craving). Similarly, Mrs. D evidences a significant response to external stimuli (other people enjoying drinking in social situations). Based on the revised information, her Risk Rating is raised to 3 (*significant risk*).

Dimension 6 (Recovery Environment) There is no change in the initial Risk Rating of 0 (*minimal or no observable risk*). AA is an increasingly meaningful support to her recovery, though she is still not as active as she planned and motivational enhancement about the level of her AA activity is indicated.

Updated Placement (Scenario 1)

The new developments and insights call for intensification of motivational enhancement strategies, which should focus on highlighting the discrepancy between Mrs. D's goal of stopping her

TABLE 7-4B

Mrs. D's Follow-up Dimensional Severity Profile: Scenario 1

	Risk Rating				
ASAM Dimension	*0 Minimal or no observable risk*	*1 Mild risk*	*2 Moderate risk*	*3 Significant risk*	*4 Severe risk*
Dimension 1: Acute Intoxication and/or Withdrawal Potential	X				
Dimension 2: Biomedical Conditions and Complications	X				
Dimension 3: Emotional, Behavioral, and Cognitive Conditions and Complications		X			
Dimension 4: Readiness to Change			X		
Dimension 5: Relapse/Continued Use/Continued Problem Potential				X	
Dimension 6: Recovery Environment	X				

problem drinking and her repeated (unsuccessful) attempts to control her drinking. Counseling should also focus on relapse prevention strategies, including forging an understanding of the circumstances surrounding her lapses, use of Cognitive-Behavioral Therapy techniques to identify the role of triggers and strategies to avoid them, and/or use of 12-step induction techniques to reemphasize Step 1 work regarding powerlessness.

If Mrs. D has not started on an antiaddiction medication, there is even more rationale now because of her continued drinking. Moreover, the newly acquired information about her positive reinforcement and reward craving may influence the choice of medication. For example, the presence of positive reinforcement and high levels of craving may favor oral or extended release injectable naltrexone. However, once again Mrs. D declined and made clear her opposition to the use of any antiaddiction medication. Further exploration of her resistance resulted in a decision to not pursue the medication option even though it was the clinician's opinion that it was the best course. Mrs. D was again encouraged to attend more meetings and to obtain even a temporary sponsor as she is invested in trying full AA involvement before considering medication at all.

The new information does not necessarily change the original placement recommendation of a Level I outpatient program, but if Mrs. D's lapses become more regular, she may need the increased monitoring and intensity of a Level II.1 intensive outpatient program.

Reassessment at Three Weeks (Scenario 2)

Mrs. D has been attending a Level I outpatient treatment program, and her work and family life are beginning to improve. However, she has lapsed over the past few days, admitting that she once again gave in to the temptation to have "just one or two." So far, she has used alcohol on three occasions, taking two drinks on two occasions and four drinks on another occasion.

As a result, she is less confident of her ability to control her drinking, but increasingly wonders again whether she might be able to manage it this time. On further discussion, she describes her lapses as often triggered by feelings of anxiety and irritability, and her idea that drinking helps her to relax. She then thinks about how much better she would feel if she could have one or two drinks. When she finally does take a drink, she feels very relieved.

Dimension 1 (Acute Intoxication/Withdrawal Potential) There is no change in the initial Risk Rating of 0 (*minimal or no observable risk*).

Dimension 2 (Biomedical Conditions and Complications) There is no change in the initial Risk Rating of 0 (*minimal or no observable risk*).

Dimension 3 (Emotional/Behavioral/Cognitive Conditions and Complications) Mrs. D evidences moderate ongoing emotional instability, as suggested by her significant anxiety and irritability and her "need" to drink to relax. This increases her Risk Rating to 2 (*moderate risk*).

Dimension 4 (Readiness to Change) Mrs. D remains motivated for treatment but is demonstrating increased ambivalence, as she begins to think that she might be able to control her drinking. This increases her Risk Rating to 2 (*moderate risk*).

Dimension 5 (Relapse/Continued Use/Continued Problem Potential) Mrs. D's lapses while in treatment raise concerns about the chronicity of her problem and her poor response to change. While her alcohol use is of moderate severity, she has been able to stop drinking in response to outside pressures (e.g., family, problems at work).

At this point, although Mrs. D's behaviors are the same as in Scenario 1, but we understand her response to substance effects differently. In Scenario 1, Mrs. D used alcohol for positive reinforcement (pleasure or reward). In Scenario 2, she describes alcohol as helping her deal with negative reinforcement (relief from the discomfort of anxiety and irritability, sometimes called relief craving). These symptoms may be persistent abstinence effects, even though Mrs. D has not reported significant acute symptoms of physiologic withdrawal. Based on this information, her Risk Rating is raised to 3 (*significant risk*).

TABLE 7-4C

Mrs. D's Follow-up Dimensional Severity Profile: Scenario 2

	Risk Rating				
ASAM Dimension	*0 Minimal or no observable risk*	*1 Mild risk*	*2 Moderate risk*	*3 Significant risk*	*4 Severe risk*
Dimension 1: Acute Intoxication and/or Withdrawal Pote ntial	X				
Dimension 2: Biomedical Conditions and Complications	X				
Dimension 3: Emotional, Behavioral, and Cognitive Conditions and Complications			X		
Dimension 4: Readiness to Change			X		
Dimension 5: Relapse/Continued Use/Continued Problem Potential				X	
Dimension 6: Recovery Environment	X				

Dimension 6 (Recovery Environment) There is no change in the initial Risk Rating of 0 (*minimal or no observable risk*). She is receiving more support from AA and now has a temporary sponsor.

Updated Placement

As in Scenario 1, the new developments and insights call for use of an antiaddiction medication. The information about the pattern of negative reinforcement and craving would influence the choice of medication. Such a situation may favor acamprosate, which may be more effective in helping Mrs. D respond to negative reinforcement. When the discussion of using an antiaddiction medication was raised, Mrs. D again made clear declined stating she did not like taking medication, wanted to do it on her own, and she was concerned that if she took the medication it would somehow devalue any resultant sobriety. After some exploratory discussion, it was decided not to aggressively pursue the use of an antiaddiction medication at this time even though the patient was an excellent candidate because of the potential damage to the therapeutic relationship but to continue motivational enhancement about its use. However, an agreement was forged between the clinician and Mrs. D that if she lapsed again, she would seriously consider the use of an antiaddiction medication. She wants to increase her AA meetings and to reach out more to her sponsor before considering medication and this was supported.

Whether the anxiety and irritability are a feature of alcohol-induced mood changes or a symptom of a co-occurring disorder, they must be addressed. If the anxiety symptoms are related to her drinking and subside with abstinence, this connection should be highlighted and used to further encourage abstinence (a motivational enhancement strategy). On the other hand, if the symptoms persist with abstinence or substantially reduced use, Mrs. D should have a psychiatric evaluation and possibly treatment for a co-occurring mental disorder.

Summary

This case illustrates rational treatment planning, following a sequence that moves first from assessment to specific treatment service needs and finally to level of care. Key factors in the assessment and placement decision include:

- The role of the following in assessing Dimension 5 relapse risk:
  - History and pattern of substance use, with a positive past response to intervention (Domain A);
  - Response to substance effects, with positive reinforcement of the pleasure of drinking, or in the alternative scenario the negative reinforcement of relieving anxiety and irritability (Domain B);
  - Response to external stimuli, with the trigger of social situations where others are drinking (Domain C); and
  - Cognitive and behavioral measures of temperament, vulnerability, and resilience, in this case marked by the patient's inappropriate overconfidence in her ability to change (Domain D).
- The rationale for choosing naltrexone in situations where the positive reinforcement of the pleasure of drinking may be salient.
- The rationale for choosing acamprosate in situations where the negative reinforcement of the relief of anxiety and irritability may be salient.

CASE 5: MR. E

Abstract

This case illustrates:

- The role of history and pattern of substance use (Domain A) in assessing Dimension 5 relapse risk.
- The use of a motivational enhancement strategies to engage the patient in treatment.
- The role of Dimension 2 medical factors in mediating Dimension 5 relapse risk.
- Considerations in selecting an antiaddiction medication for a patient who has impaired liver and kidney function.

Initial Presentation

Mr. E, a 55-year-old man, has been a patient of yours for a number of years. He is alcohol-dependent with associated impairment. He has been intermittently involved in psychosocial treatments, with only transient partial success.

Mr. E is willing to try to reduce his drinking, but is not interested in abstinence. He claims he would be "fine" if he cut down and adds: "there's nothing wrong with a drink before dinner and a glass of wine with dinner." He has failed previous attempts to quit or to adhere to the limits he set for himself, with the result that his marriage is at risk of imminent failure.

Initial Assessment

Dimension 1 (Acute Intoxication/Withdrawal Potential) The available information does not indicate a problem in this Dimension, leading to an initial Risk Rating of 0 (*minimal or no observable risk*).

Dimension 2 (Biomedical Conditions and Complications) The available information does not indicate a problem in this Dimension, leading to an initial Risk Rating of 0 (*minimal or no observable risk*).

Dimension 3 (Emotional/Behavioral/Cognitive Conditions and Complications) Mr. E is struggling with the potential failure of his marriage. Therefore, his initial Risk Rating is 2 (*moderate risk*).

Dimension 4 (Readiness to Change) Mr. E is in the Precontemplation Stage of Change for abstinence but in the Preparation Stage for reducing his drinking. Based on multiple failed attempts to change using similar self-direction of personal resources in the past, as well as his lack of engagement in treatment, Mr. E's initial Risk Rating is 3 (*significant risk*).

Dimension 5 (Relapse/Continued Use/Continued Problem Potential) Mr. E's pattern of alcohol use is of significant chronicity and severity, without sustained abstinence. He has shown a poor response to previous psychosocial treatments and other motivators of change, as demonstrated by his failed previous attempts to quit or to adhere to the limits he set for himself. Complicating the situation is the imminent collapse of his marriage because of his drinking.

We have no information about his response to substance effects or to external stimuli. In terms of temperament, vulnerabilities, and resilience (Domain D), the patient seems to have poor coping skills and a very unrealistic level of confidence in his ability to self-direct change. His inability to learn from past unsuccessful efforts to limit his drinking and other assessment information lead to an initial Risk Rating of 3 (*significant risk*).

Dimension 6 (Recovery Environment) If Mr. E's marriage fails, his recovery supports are uncertain. Therefore, his initial Risk Rating is at least 1 (*mild risk*).

Initial Placement

Mr. E. expresses a readiness to change by cutting down or controlling his drinking, although he has not yet learned from previous experience that he is unable to do so. He seems ready to

TABLE 7-5A

Mr. E's Initial Dimensional Severity Profile

	Risk Rating				
ASAM Dimension	*0 Minimal or no observable risk*	*1 Mild Risk*	*2 Moderate Risk*	*3 Significant Risk*	*4 Severe Risk*
Dimension 1: Acute Intoxication and/or Withdrawal Potential	X				
Dimension 2: Biomedical Conditions and Complications	X				
Dimension 3: Emotional, Behavioral, and Cognitive Conditions and Complications			X		
Dimension 4: Readiness to Change				X	
Dimension 5: Relapse/Continued Use/Continued Problem Potential				X	
Dimension 6: Recovery Environment		X			

accept assistance toward that goal, but not (yet) toward the goal of abstinence. If he is unable or unwilling to understand or accept his loss of control over alcohol, an appropriate motivational enhancement strategy would be to engage him in his initial goal of cutting down, while providing monitoring of and feedback on his success or lack thereof. An overly confrontational or premature insistence on abstinence may lead to premature treatment termination, whereas treatment retention should be a paramount goal. The emphasis should be placed on motivational enhancement strategies targeted to help the patient understand the discrepancy between his stated goal of improving his psychosocial function (e.g., his marriage) and his inability to control his drinking.

Mr. E is an excellent candidate for antiaddiction medication as an adjunct to psychosocial treatment. Such medication could be offered as part of an engagement/ motivational strategy, by explaining to Mr. E that it may help him to successfully cut down, although the overall goal is for the medication to help him achieve abstinence. Even if Mr. E does not achieve total abstinence, any reduction in his drinking will be helpful. The patient probably is not a good candidate for disulfiram because of his stated intention to continue drinking. His lack of motivation to achieve abstinence may favor oral or long-acting injectable naltrexone. It may be constructive to consider an analogy to a patient with Type I diabetes, who is willing to take insulin but says he is unable to adhere to his diet despite obesity, carbohydrate binging, and acknowledging that he ought to "cut down" on sweets. In this case, we would continue to work on engagement and motivational enhancement to achieve the desired change in the patient's behavior, but not refuse to prescribe medication or to continue care.

Mr. E should be placed in a Level II.1 IOP program, but may alternatively be managed in a Level I outpatient treatment program with higher than "average" intensity (one that meets more than once per week or and/or has more than one service hour per contact) and/or with "extra" supports. Such a program, with intensity somewhere between Level I and Level II.1, while officially falling within the range of Level I, might be unofficially construed as a Level I.5 program. The decision between Level I and Level II.1 would be based in large part on his personal choice, motivation, availability, and logistics, and his perception of the balance of the benefits versus the treatment burden of the intensity of a proposed IOP placement. Extra supports could include a recommendation for participation in a self-help recovery group, a recommendation for family counseling, and/or participation by his wife in the monitoring of his medication treatment. Participation in Al-Anon should be suggested to his wife as part of the plan. If he does not show evidence of improvement in a relatively short time in a Level I program, then the indication for Level II.1 increases.

Initial Presentation (Scenario 2)

In this alternative scenario, Mr. E's laboratory results show moderately elevated liver enzymes. The initial presentation is otherwise unchanged as above.

Dimension 1 (Acute Intoxication/Withdrawal Potential) There is no change in the initial Risk Rating of 0 (*minimal or no observable risk*).

Dimension 2 (Biomedical Conditions and Complications) The change in laboratory values leads to an increase in Mr. E's Risk Rating to 2 (*moderate risk*).

Dimension 3 (Emotional/Behavioral/Cognitive Conditions and Complications) There is no change in the initial Risk Rating of 2 (*moderate risk*).

Dimension 4 (Readiness to Change) There is no change in the initial Risk Rating of 3 (*significant risk*).

Dimension 5 (Relapse/Continued Use/Continued Problem Potential) There is no change in the initial Risk Rating of 3 (*significant risk*).

Dimension 6 (Recovery Environment) There is no change in the initial Risk Rating of 1 (*mild risk*).

Initial Placement (Scenario 2)

Because of the increased risk of biomedical problems in Dimension 2, the consequences of relapse are more severe, the indication for a higher intensity of counseling is even stronger. If he is judged likely to be responsive, he would benefit from placement in a Level II.1 intensive outpatient program. The indication for an antiaddiction medication is also stronger. Also, the physiologic evidence of alcohol's effects on Mr. E's liver function should be used to enhance his motivation toward sobriety.

However, the evidence of severe hepatocellular injury is a relative contraindication to naltrexone, in that the reported association between naltrexone and liver toxicity has raised concerns that the drug should not be used in the presence of existing liver damage. However because alcohol is more toxic to the liver than naltrexone and the potential benefits of reduced alcohol consumption outweigh the risks of naltrexone, improving liver function tests would favor initiation or continuation of treatment with naltrexone, accompanied by ongoing monitoring of liver function. If testing shows liver enzymes at a level more than 4 to 5 times higher than the normal range, naltrexone should be discontinued or not initiated.

Acamprosate does not raise similar concerns about effect on liver function. In situations where naltrexone is considered problematic because of liver toxicity, acamprosate is a good alternative. Additionally, the patient needs medical follow-up for his abnormal liver function tests.

The patient definitely needs work to enhance his medication adherence. Adherence should be explicitly encouraged and monitored by the counseling staff and should become a focus of the treatment plan. If Mr. E is motivated by his wife's concern, it would probably be productive to involve her in helping with medication adherence. For example, she could collaborate by monitoring and tracking his self-administration of the medication. The details of that arrangement should be negotiated—whether she will remind him, which may be beneficial because she may be more motivated to "remember," but also could be detrimental if he perceives it as "nagging" and it thus becomes an increased source of conflict or whether she will only observe and report back to the treatment team (this may be beneficial in promoting his responsibility and autonomy but is a less active intervention).

Initial Presentation (Scenario 3)

In this alternative scenario, Mr. E's medical history and laboratory results reflect impaired renal (kidney) function. The initial presentation is otherwise unchanged as above.

Dimension 1 (Acute Intoxication/Withdrawal Potential) There is no change in the initial Risk Rating of 0 (*minimal or no observable risk*).

Dimension 2 (Biomedical Conditions and Complications) The change in laboratory values leads to an increase in Mr. E's Risk Rating to 2 (*moderate risk*).

Dimension 3 (Emotional/Behavioral/Cognitive Conditions and Complications) There is no change in the initial Risk Rating of 2 (*moderate risk*).

Dimension 4 (Readiness to Change) There is no change in the initial Risk Rating of 3 (*significant risk*).

TABLE 7-5B

Mr. E's Initial Dimensional Severity Profile: Scenario 2

	Risk Rating				
ASAM Dimension	*0 Minimal or no observable risk*	*1 Mild risk*	*2 Moderate risk*	*3 Significant risk*	*4 Severe risk*
Dimension 1: Acute Intoxication and/or Withdrawal Pote ntial	X				
Dimension 2: Biomedical Conditions and Complications			X		
Dimension 3: Emotional, Behavioral, and Cognitive Conditions and Complications			X		
Dimension 4: Readiness to Change				X	
Dimension 5: Relapse/Continued Use/Continued Problem Potential				X	
Dimension 6: Recovery Environment		X			

Dimension 5 (Relapse/Continued Use/Continued Problem Potential) There is no change in the initial Risk Rating of 3 (*significant risk*).

Dimension 6 (Recovery Environment) There is no change in the initial Risk Rating of 1 (*mild risk*).

Initial Placement (Scenario 3)

The only difference in the treatment plan from that discussed in Scenario 1 is in medication management. If Mr. E was on acamprosate, the acamprosate dose must be adjusted for renal insufficiency. On the other hand, increased creatinine levels do not require any change if the patient is taking naltrexone. Additionally, the patient needs medical follow-up for his abnormal renal function.

TABLE 7-5C

Mr. E's Initial Dimensional Severity Profile: Scenario 3

ASAM Dimension	*Risk Rating* 0 Minimal or no observable risk	1 Mild risk	2 Moderate risk	3 Significant risk	4 Severe risk
Dimension 1: Acute Intoxication and/or Withdrawal Potential	X				
Dimension 2: Biomedical Conditions and Complications			X		
Dimension 3: Emotional, Behavioral, and Cognitive Conditions and Complications			X		
Dimension 4: Readiness to Change				X	
Dimension 5: Relapse/Continued Use/Continued Problem Potential				X	
Dimension 6: Recovery Environment		X			

Reassessment at Four Weeks

At a follow-up visit 4 weeks later, treatment with an antiaddiction medication has not been initiated. Mr. E discloses that he has not been able to stop drinking for more than one day at a time and is experiencing moderate withdrawal symptoms.

Dimension 1 (Acute Intoxication/Withdrawal Potential) The Risk Rating is raised to 2 (*moderate risk*) because of Mr. E's withdrawal symptoms.

Dimension 2 (Biomedical Conditions and Complications) The change in laboratory values leads to an increase in Mr. E's Risk Rating to 2 (*moderate risk*).

Dimension 3 (Emotional/Behavioral/Cognitive Conditions and Complications) There is no change in the initial Risk Rating of 2 (*moderate risk*).

Dimension 4 (Readiness to Change) There is no change in the initial Risk Rating of 3 (*significant risk*).

Dimension 5 (Relapse/Continued Use/Continued Problem Potential) There is no change in the initial Risk Rating of 3 (*significant risk*).

Dimension 6 (Recovery Environment) There is no change in the initial Risk Rating of 1 (*mild risk*).

Updated Placement

Mr. E needs detoxification services. Additionally, the initiation of antiaddiction pharmacotherapy after 3 to 4 days of abstinence is indicated.

TABLE 7-5D

Mr. E's Dimensional Severity Profile at Follow-Up

	Risk Rating				
ASAM Dimension	*0 Stable (no observable risk)*	*1 Mild risk*	*2 Moderate risk*	*3 Significant risk*	*4 Severe risk*
Dimension 1: Acute Intoxication and/or Withdrawal Potential			X		
Dimension 2: Biomedical Conditions and Complications			X		
Dimension 3: Emotional, Behavioral, and Cognitive Conditions and Complications			X		
Dimension 4: Readiness to Change				X	
Dimension 5: Relapse/Continued Use/Continued Problem Potential				X	
Dimension 6: Recovery Environment		X			

For detoxification, consider the possibility of placing the patient in an ambulatory setting (e.g., a Level II.5-D program), but given the interaction with Dimensions 4 and 5 and the need to support his induction into pharmacotherapy, placement in a Level III.7-D (Medically Monitored Detoxification) program may be appropriate, if the patient agrees.

Summary

This case illustrates rational treatment planning, following a sequence that moves first from assessment to specific treatment service needs, and finally to level of care. It also addresses the interaction between impairments in liver and kidney function and the decision to use a specific antiaddiction medication.

CASE 6: MS. F

Abstract

Key factors in this case are:

- Use of a motivational enhancement strategy to engage the patient in treatment.
- Use of external leverage as a treatment engagement strategy.
- The rationale for a decision to use an antiaddiction medication to treat alcohol abuse (as opposed to dependence).
- Initial treatment in a physician's office practice rather than a formal specialty addiction treatment program

Initial Presentation

Ms. F, a 27-year-old woman with a 4-year-old son, has been referred by a child welfare worker because of neglect related to problem drinking. Her goal is to retain custody of her son.

The patient acknowledges that she does drink, "partying" on the weekends, and that she has "maybe made some bad choices." But she denies that she has a "problem" with alcohol, and insists that she could stop drinking if she wanted to do so. She adds that she is willing to take an antiaddiction medication in order to comply with the child welfare case plan, but she adamantly refuses to participate in a formal treatment program with "those drunks and junkies." She resists all efforts to persuade her to try counseling, self-help groups, or other psychosocial interventions.

Initial Assessment

Dimension 1 (Acute Intoxication/Withdrawal Potential) The available information does not indicate a problem in this Dimension, leading to an initial Risk Rating of 0 (*minimal or no observable risk*).

Dimension 2 (Biomedical Conditions and Complications) The available information does not indicate a problem in this Dimension, leading to an initial Risk Rating of 0 (*minimal or no observable risk*).

Dimension 3 (Emotional/Behavioral/Cognitive Conditions and Complications) The available information does not indicate a problem in this Dimension, leading to an initial Risk Rating of 0 (*minimal or no observable risk*).

Dimension 4 (Readiness to Change) Ms. F is in a Precontemplation Stage of Change with regard to whether she has a problem with alcohol, but she is in the Action Stage regarding her motivation to retain custody of her child. This leads her to the Preparation Stage of Change with regard to taking antiaddiction medication. However, she is in a Precontemplation Stage about entering psychosocial substance abuse treatment. Because of her desire to retain custody of her son, she is willing to partially adhere to *some* treatment recommendations. This results in an initial Risk Rating of 3 (*significant risk*).

Dimension 5 (Relapse/Continued Use/Continued Problem Potential) While there is little specific information, we will assume that the child welfare caseworker's conclusions are accurate and that there is moderate chronicity and severity. Moreover, Ms. F's denial of her alcohol problem increases the risk of continued use. Therefore, her initial Risk Rating is 2 (*moderate risk*).

Dimension 6 (Recovery Environment) The available information about Ms. F's status in Dimension 6 is that she will lose custody of her son if she fails to address her drinking. This is the major factor motivating her toward change. Therefore, her initial Risk Rating is 2 (*moderate risk*).

Initial Placement

Psychosocial treatment is clearly indicated. Although the patient refuses the recommended treatment plan, it is not helpful to withhold treatment entirely. Instead, the appropriate strategy is to continue to see her as an office patient (usually something less formal and intensive than a specialty addiction Level I outpatient program); to agree to prescribe an antiaddiction medication (acamprosate or oral or long-acting injectable naltrexone, or disulfiram); to monitor her use of and response to the medication; to continue to educate her about alcohol use disorders in an effort to raise her problem self-recognition; and to employ motivational enhancement strategies to overcome her resistance to change beyond trying to retain custody of her son.

Given her current attitude, insisting on specialty psychosocial treatment as a condition for continued treatment risks losing the relationship and the motivation that currently exists. Therefore, it may be wise to make prescribing the medication contingent on office visits with continued engagement motivational enhancement strategies. It may be useful to propose that Ms. F try to stop drinking without additional formal psychosocial treatment, with the suggestion that she might reconsider such treatment if she is unable to stop on her own. Consideration also should be given to asking her to go to one or two self-help recovery group meetings to learn more about alcohol problems. It is instructive to consider an analogy to a patient with hypertension, who agrees to take antihypertensive medication but refused to alter her lifestyle, which involves a high-sodium diet, smoking, and no exercise. In this case, while we would continue to work on engagement and motivational enhancement toward behavioral change, we would not refuse to prescribe medicine or continue care based on her lack of commitment to behavioral change. In contrast, some addiction treatment practitioners might refuse to care for a patient who is considered noncompliant or "not ready" for treatment.

TABLE 7-6A

Ms. F's Initial Dimensional Severity Profile

ASAM Dimension	*Risk Rating* *0 Minimal or no observable risk*	*1 Mild risk*	*2 Moderate risk*	*3 Significant risk*	*4 Severe risk*
Dimension 1: Acute Intoxication and/or Withdrawal Potential	X				
Dimension 2: Biomedical Conditions and Complications	X				
Dimension 3: Emotional, Behavioral, and Cognitive Conditions and Complications	X				
Dimension 4: Readiness to Change				X	
Dimension 5: Relapse/Continued Use/Continued Problem Potential			X		
Dimension 6: Recovery Environment			X		

Reassessment at Six Weeks

At a follow-up visit, the information gathered suggests a significant pattern of alcohol abuse, marked by sporadic binges and considerable impairment. Evidence includes two citations for driving under the influence (DUI) and at least one emergency department visit for alcohol-related trauma. However, Ms. F does not meet the *DSM* criteria for alcohol dependence.

Updated Placement

The additional information suggests increased risk in Dimension 5, which is upgraded to a Risk Rating of 3 (*significant risk*).

Ms. F is now a candidate for a Level II.1 intensive outpatient program, but she continues to refuse formal substance abuse treatment. It may be useful to recommend that her continued custody of her son be contingent on her participation in psychosocial treatment (either initially or if she does not make suitable progress). It may be suitable to add criminal justice leverage if the DUI arrests provide additional tools for engagement or external motivation.

Given the potential that Ms. F's current use of alcohol will lead to serious harm to herself or others, as well as her potential motivation for adherence, consider switching to or adding disulfiram, linking medication supervision and adherence to the recommended terms of the child welfare case.

The formal indications for pharmacotherapy for alcohol use disorders are for alcohol *dependence* rather than alcohol *abuse*. Nevertheless, given the significant consequences for some patients, many experts recommend use of an antiaddiction medication in such cases to help the patient achieve a reduction in his or her alcohol use and as a motivational tool toward abstinence and recovery.

Summary

This case illustrates rational treatment planning, following a sequence that moves first from assessment to specific treatment service needs, and finally to level of care. It features the use of a motivational enhancement technique (i.e., accepting a trial of the patient's self-selected plan to take medication but not to attend psychosocial treatment) as a strategy to engage the patient in treatment.

CASE 7: MR. G

Abstract

This case illustrates:

- An example of ambulatory detoxification and transition into IOP rehabilitation in a case of high risk of withdrawal.
- The role of recovery environment (Dimension 6) in determining the treatment plan and placement decisions.

Initial Presentation

Mr. G is a 43-year-old man who was referred by his primary physician after a physical examination had revealed elevated liver enzymes (AST = 90, ALT = 60, GGT = 110). The physician had been cautioning the patient for several years about his excessive drinking, focusing particularly on the negative effect that this was having on the patient's hypertension, which had been poorly controlled despite taking the antihypertensive medication atenolol. The patient acknowledged morning drinking to relieve tremulousness. He rejected his physician's recommendation for hospitalization for detoxification but was willing to accept a referral for an outpatient evaluation.

Mr. G arrived for his 9 a.m. appointment, accompanied by his wife. She had been in his company for the previous 10 hours and supported his assertion that he had had no alcohol since 11 p.m. the night before, in accordance with the instructions he had received when he had made his appointment. The patient described drinking on a daily basis for most of the past 4 years. For the past year his drinking began in the morning and he averaged one fifth of vodka daily. When he had tried to stop drinking on his own, he would become tremulous. In response to specific questioning, he acknowledged that he had experienced a grand mal withdrawal seizure 6 months previously and had not disclosed this to his primary physician. He denied any history of withdrawal hallucinations. His medical history was notable for his hypertension and alcoholic hepatitis but otherwise negative. He had no history of significant mood swings.

On examination, he interacted appropriately and cooperatively. He described himself as feeling "shaky." His blood alcohol level (BAL) as measured by breath analyzer was 0.12 mg%. His blood pressure was 150/100, his pulse was 92, and he was afebrile. His sclerae were nonicteric. His hands at rest had a fine tremor, which intensified to moderate when his arms were extended. His anxiety was moderately severe and he felt mildly depressed. No gross abnormalities were detected on mental status. His mini-mental status exam (MMSE) score was 28/30. His CIWA-Ar score was 16.

He stated that he knew that he had a problem with alcohol that he had not been able to deal with successfully on his own. He had attended a few meetings of AA but had not found one with which he was comfortable. His drinking had become increasingly solitary. He believed that he had successfully hidden his problem from friends and work—which was supported by his wife.

His wife stated that their marriage of 10 years had become strained as a result of his drinking, but she had not seriously considered separation. Her own drinking pattern had been a glass of wine every 1 to 2 days. She was willing to cooperate with removing all alcohol from the house. She revealed that she had been attending Al-Anon meetings for the past 6 months and had found them to be useful. The patient accepted the recommendation for detoxification, but again elected not to go into a residential program. When an alternative treatment plan for intensive outpatient detoxification and rehabilitation was described to him, he was able to understand it and made a commitment to adhere to the instructions that he received. His wife was willing to return in the evening to drive the patient home and also agreed to attend a once weekly group for relatives at the program.

Dimensional Assessment

Dimension 1 (Acute Intoxication/Withdrawal Potential) The pattern of heavy drinking throughout the day, his past history of a withdrawal seizure, and his CIWA-Ar score of 16 give Mr. G a Risk Rating of 3 (*significant risk*).

Dimension 2 (Biomedical Conditions and Complications) Mr. G's hypertension has probably not been adequately controlled because of the heavy alcohol intake. Given the involvement of his physician, the removal of alcohol should make his hypertension manageable, giving him a Risk Rating of 1 (*mild risk*).

Dimension 3 (Emotional/Behavioral/Cognitive Conditions and Complications) Mr. G has had no history of psychiatric symptoms. His mild depression at presentation will probably resolve spontaneously with treatment of his alcohol dependence. This suggests a Risk Rating of 1 (*mild risk*) in this Dimension.

Dimension 4 (Readiness to Change) Mr. G appears to be on his way toward accepting the existence of his alcoholism. Acknowledging his unsuccessful attempts to deal with the problem on

TABLE 7-7A

Mr. G's Initial Dimensional Severity Profile

	Risk Rating				
ASAM Dimension	*0 Minimal or no observable risk*	*1 Mild risk*	*2 Moderate risk*	*3 Significant risk*	*4 Severe risk*
Dimension 1: Acute Intoxication and/or Withdrawal Potential				X	
Dimension 2: Biomedical Conditions and Complications		X			
Dimension 3: Emotional, Behavioral, and Cognitive Conditions and Complications		X			
Dimension 4: Readiness to Change			X		
Dimension 5: Relapse/Continued Use/Continued Problem Potential				X	
Dimension 6: Recovery Environment		X			

his own and his having accepted his physician's referral indicates that he is ready to accept outside help with it. He is in the early Action stage of change. On the other hand, he has no previous experience with treatment and his initial encounters with AA were not positive. Therefore, his Risk Rating in Dimension 4 is 2 (*moderate risk*).

Dimension 5 (Relapse/Continued Use/Continued Problem Potential) Mr. G has not had any periods of sustained abstinence. He has had significant negative reinforcement and cravings, frequently drinking to alleviate withdrawal symptoms. Given how extensive his daily drinking has been, he will have to reestablish almost entire new daily routines to establish sobriety. He can be expected to experience ongoing cravings and will need to be oriented to the concept of triggers. This combination would merit a Risk Rating of 3 (*significant risk*).

Dimension 6 (Recovery Environment) Mr. G is fortunate to have a supportive, nonalcoholic spouse. Although his drinking has been heavy and steady, he has not developed social group to support it. His attempts at AA involvement, while not successful, suggest a base of relative openness from which to work. Therefore, his severity in this Dimension justifies a Risk Rating of 1 (*mild risk*).

Placement and Discussion

The severity of Mr. G's physical addiction and withdrawal potential would have justified admission to a Level III.7-D, medically monitored inpatient detoxification service. Because his medical and psychiatric complications were minimal, his level of cooperation was adequate, and his recovery environment was supportive, treatment in a Level II.D: Ambulatory Detoxification With Extended Onsite Monitoring was an acceptable alternative when the patient refused inpatient admission. The intensity of medical services and monitoring delivered in the PHP setting described below the patient's level of commitment and adherence, and the level of family support allow safe ambulatory detoxification with a fairly high level of withdrawal severity (Dimension 1, Risk Rating 3). A significant worsening of any of these factors would require transferring him to an inpatient setting to complete his detoxification.

Mr. G was given 50 mg chlordiazepoxide orally. One hour later, he reported persistent "shakiness" with no subjective effect from the medication, and was given another 50 mg. Thirty minutes later, he reported beginning to less "shaky" and agreed to sit in a group in the intensive outpatient/partial hospital rehabilitation program. He continued to receive 50 mg of chlordiazepoxide each hour, for a total of 200 mg. At 1 p.m., his BAL was 0.04 mg%, his blood pressure was 140/92, his pulse was 76, and his CIWA-Ar score was 9. His tremor had decreased from moderate to mild. He described himself as feeling tired and went to sleep for 1 hour. When he awoke, his anxiety had returned. He was given another 50 mg chlordiazepoxide and his symptoms subsided. At 4 p.m. his BAL was zero and he was given 125 mg of disulfiram.

By 6 p.m., no withdrawal symptoms had recurred. He was given a supply of three 50 mg doses of chlordiazepoxide to take home, and instructed to take 50 mg at bedtime and repeat this every hour until he fell asleep or if he awakened during the night.

He returned the next morning, having been driven by his wife, and reported that he had fallen asleep after taking 2 doses of 50 mg chlordiazepoxide. He had awakened during the night, taken the last 50 mg and had slept through the rest of the night. His BAL was 0, his blood pressure was 136/90, his pulse was 72, and his CIWA-Ar score was 12. He complained of feeling anxious and he still had a mild tremor of his hands. He was given another 50 mg of chlordiazepoxide that eliminated his anxiety and reduced his tremor. He was also given 125 mg of disulfiram. He participated in the IOP/PHP for the second time and was given 2 doses of 50 mg chlordiazepoxide to take home with instructions to take one dose at bedtime and the second dose after an hour if needed for sleep.

On the third day, he drove himself to the facility and reported that he had slept through the night on the first dose of 50 mg chlordiazepoxide. His BAL was 0, his blood pressure was 134/90, his pulse was 70, and his CIWA-Ar score was 6. He still had a mild tremor but was not anxious. He was told that the tremor would resolve on its own over a period of days and that no more medication would be given for this. He was given another 125 mg of disulfiram and was instructed to take the unused 50 mg of chlordiazepoxide for sleep if needed, but to bring it back to the facility if he did not use it.

The next day, he reported sleeping through the night without the chlordiazepoxide, which he returned. On that and every subsequent visit he was given 125 mg of disulfiram but no more chlordiazepoxide. His tremor resolved after the seventh day.

During the second week of treatment, he reported hypersomnia, taking naps during the afternoon and sleeping through his alarm in the morning, both of which were unusual for him. He was given reassurance that these symptoms would subside without specific intervention. He was pleased and surprised to find that his energy, productivity, mood, and physical sense of well-being were greater than it had been than in any time in recent memory. He no longer felt depressed and reported no cravings for alcohol, but found that he had an unusual craving for ice cream. He felt very confident that his "drinking days are done" and questioned whether he really needed to continue with treatment at such a high level of intensity. On the other hand, he acknowledged that he sometimes had thoughts that since he now felt stronger, he might be able to drink in moderation. He attended an AA meeting and reported that he felt uncomfortable with references in the meeting to a "Higher Power" and the fact that at the end of the meeting everyone held hands and said the Lord's Prayer. His wife attended the relatives' group and participated appropriately. She also maintained her attendance at Al-Anon.

A "front loaded" symptom-triggered detoxification protocol was followed, using a long-acting benzodiazepine. Such an approach allows the patient to achieve rapid comfort and safety while ultimately using less medication than a time-driven protocol. The use of a long-acting benzodiazepine provides better protection from seizures and less likelihood of later symptom rebound after being tapered, than does the more widely used short-acting agents lorazepam and oxazepam. The presence of mildly increased liver enzymes is no reason to avoid detoxifying agents that are metabolized by the liver. The only adjustment is that lower doses of the medication may be necessary. The onset of action of chlordiazepoxide is sufficiently rapid to protect the patient from a further progression of the withdrawal syndrome.

Detoxification and rehabilitation services have traditionally been separated from one another, sometimes leading to treatment being foreshortened when the now comfortable detoxified patient chooses not to follow through with ongoing treatment. Now that detoxification techniques have improved significantly, this separation is no longer necessary if a program is structured so as to allow participation in both simultaneously. The patient's cognitive functioning during withdrawal/detoxification may in fact not allow him to get the full benefit of the rehabilitation program. However, the treatment engagement, including the interpersonal bonds formed with the rehabilitation clinicians and the other patients in the program can create an essential bridge to increase the likelihood that the patient will follow through with the treatment necessary for a solid recovery.

Because of his significant relapse risk (Dimension 5, Risk Rating 3) pharmacotherapy is very strongly recommended for relapse prevention, as part of his comprehensive treatment plan. Induction onto disulfiram early in treatment during the detoxification phase adds additional protection during this very vulnerable period. Disulfiram should always be used with adherence/compliance enhancement procedures. In the IOP setting this can include supervised administration of medication, along with group observation for additional reinforcement through ritual and peer pressure and support. Additionally, introduction early in treatment may further reinforce medication adherence.

Acamprosate would also be a reasonable alternative in this case, especially during a period of persistent subacute abstinence symptoms with a history of relapse partially driven by negative reinforcement.

Upon Completion of Detoxification: Reassessment

After the acute phase of detoxification has been completed, the patient experienced a residual tremor that was not medicated in order to reduce the likelihood of cross addiction. The patient experienced the protracted withdrawal symptom of excessive sleepiness, which again was not treated with medication. Following this, the patient experienced a mild euphoria in the context of the newly experienced benefits of initial abstinence, commonly know as a "pink cloud." Although not invariable, it occurs frequently and may be as brief as a few days or may persist for a few weeks. The best approach is to allow the patient to enjoy this period, but to make clear that it is transient, so that the patient is not unduly disappointed when it inevitably ends.

Dimension 1 The acute discomfort as well as the danger of the withdrawal syndrome has passed. The Risk Rating has improved to 0 (*minimal or no observable risk*).

Dimension 2 The patient's blood pressure has improved, but is still elevated. It will still need to be monitored and treated. After several months, the absence of alcohol may lead to a reduction in blood pressure so that antihypertensive medication may need to be reduced or even eliminated. The Risk Rating remains at 1 (*mild*).

Dimension 3 (Emotional/Behavioral/Cognitive Conditions and Complications) Depressive symptoms are no longer present. The Risk Rating has decreased to 0 (*minimal or no observable risk*).

Dimensions 4, 5, and 6 Although the patient made excellent progress and his wife followed through on her commitment to participate, it is too early to reduce the risk rating in any of these dimensions.

Dimension 5 His acute risk of relapse is somewhat alleviated by attenuation of withdrawal symptoms and by induction onto pharmacotherapy with disulfiram. On the other hand his mild euphoria of initial abstinence (commonly called "pink cloud") may lead to a false sense of confidence, with possible decreased treatment engagement and/or temptation to test loss of control. On balance, his Risk Rating remains significant at 3.

Placement and Discussion

The patient will continue to participate in the IOP, followed by Continued Care at a Level I treatment level. His difficulties with AA will be addressed on an ongoing basis. Suggestions for

TABLE 7-7B

Mr. G's Postdetoxification Dimensional Severity Profile

	Risk Rating				
ASAM Dimension	*0* *Minimal or no observable risk*	*1* *Mild risk*	*2* *Moderate risk*	*3* *Significant risk*	*4* *Severe risk*
Dimension 1: Acute Intoxication and/or Withdrawal Potential	X				
Dimension 2: Biomedical Conditions and Complications		X			
Dimension 3: Emotional, Behavioral, and Cognitive Conditions and Complications	X				
Dimension 4: Readiness to Change			X		
Dimension 5: Relapse/Continued Use/Continued Problem Potential			X		
Dimension 6: Recovery Environment		X			

compatible groups will be made and the possibility of participating in a secular support group such as Smart Recovery will be made.

Summary

This case illustrates how a patient with a very high risk for withdrawal can be well managed on an ambulatory basis if he is sufficiently cooperative and his environment is supportive.

APPENDIX A

Assessment Process and Instruments

Formal assessment provides the standardization and credibility necessary for effective treatment matching, which is a critical step in overall treatment planning. The data-gathering processes involved in a clinical assessment can promote behavioral change by allowing detailed objective feedback to the patient about his or her behaviors, symptoms, and consequences. Sometimes the objective interview process itself may help the patient to move from the precontemplation stage to the contemplation stage (during which he or she becomes aware of the need to change).

Assessment instruments offer several advantages over the conventional clinical interviews for both treatment matching and treatment planning. A valid instrument offers a uniform inquiry, comprehensive coverage of essential areas, quantification of data, and standardization of the interpretations of the data. What is clear is that there are significant clinical advantages to quantifying the alcohol withdrawal syndrome. By identifying patients who require pharmacotherapies, while sparing the majority of patients whose syndromes are not so severe, use of assessment instruments can help the clinician avoid over- or undertreatment.

Assessments without instruments cannot provide these features, because interviewers may vary widely in style (e.g., use of open versus closed-ended questions), areas of inquiry (severity of substance dependence versus psychopathology), depth of inquiry (screening superficially in some areas versus detailed probing in others), units of measure (severity of drug use may be measured in terms of quantity, frequency, recency, and/or expenditures), and—most importantly—interviewers may vary widely in the assumptions they use in interpreting assessment results.

CHARACTERISTICS OF VALID ASSESSMENT INSTRUMENTS

An assessment instrument should demonstrate certain psychometric properties if it is to be accepted for clinical research or routine clinical use. The items that make up the instrument should have clear meanings, should be distinct and parsimonious (i.e., nonredundant), and should relate to one another in a coherent way (e.g., items that are logically connected should be grouped with one another in subscales). Different raters should be able to use the instrument and obtain similar ratings (inter-rater reliability) and the same patient should obtain similar results on two different, closely spaced administrations (test-retest reliability).

In addition to reliability, an instrument must have demonstrated validity. The instrument and its items should be based on an underlying logical framework, or construct. The instrument should make sense as an effort to assess the intended area; that is, it should demonstrate face validity. If an accepted "gold standard" measure exists, a comparative trial between the two instruments should yield similar results, demonstrating convergent validity. Different scores should distinguish different outcomes, demonstrating predictive validity. Finally, the instrument should obtain different results from those of another instrument designed for a different purpose (discriminant validity).

INSTRUMENTS FOR USE IN STANDARDIZED ASSESSMENTS

While many measures exist, the instruments described here have been selected for their utility in treatment matching and treatment planning, their strong psychometric properties (reliability and validity), and the availability of data on their use. What follows is the description of a set of instruments that incorporates these principles and that provides a comprehensive assessment capable of yielding sufficient information for treatment matching and/or treatment planning.

Instruments may be combined to create a comprehensive battery that yields data for matching patients to levels of care.

Addiction Severity Index

The Addiction Severity Index (ASI) is a widely used semistructured interview that is designed to elicit information about areas of the patient's life that may contribute to and/or be affected by his or her substance use problem. The ASI assesses seven dimensions that typically are of foremost concern to patients with substance dependence. These are: Medical Status, Employment/Support Status, Drug/Alcohol Use, Legal Status, Family History, Family/Social Relationships, and Psychiatric Status.

The ASI asks factual questions about the amount of alcohol and drug use within the preceding 30 days, as well as lifetime use; about living arrangements, and disruptions in relationships; and the number of legal charges resulting in convictions.

A potentially useful feature of the ASI is that it first establishes with the patient a detailed list of adverse behaviors and consequences of addiction. Then, having acknowledged these consequences, the patient is asked to assess the severity of his or her problems in each area. A Severity Rating Scale asks "How important to you now is treatment for these alcohol problems?" on a 5-point scale, with potential responses ranging from "not at all important" to "extremely important."

The ASI is designed to be administered by a trained technician and in approximately 40 minutes to 1 hour. It also is available in a self-administered, computerized format. A smaller subset of items is used in follow-up interviews to assess the patient's progress over time. The ASI can be administered as frequently as once a month to assess serial change.

Alcohol Dependence Scale

The Alcohol Dependence Scale (ADS) provides a quantitative measure of the severity of alcohol dependence consistent with the concept of the alcohol dependence syndrome.

Because the test can be administered in approximately 5 minutes, it can be used in a variety of settings. The ADS also is widely used as a research and clinical tool (Skinner & Allen, 1982).

The 25 items cover alcohol withdrawal symptoms, impaired control over drinking, awareness of a compulsion to drink, increased tolerance to alcohol, and salience of alcohol-seeking behavior (Skinner & Horn, 1984). The ADS has been used primarily for assessment of adults in treatment settings; however, researchers also have used the instrument in general population and correctional settings.

The ADS has been found to have excellent predictive value with respect to a *DSM-IV* diagnosis. Moreover, the ADS yields a measure of the severity of dependence that is important in treatment planning, especially with respect to the intensity of care (Allen & Columbus, 1995).

The printed instructions for the ADS refer to the preceding 12-month period. However, instructions can be altered for use as an outcome measure at selected intervals (e.g., at 6, 12, or 24 months) following treatment. The ADS has been found to be reliable and valid. Research shows that it has excellent predictive value with respect to *DSM* diagnoses (Allen & Columbus, 1995).

The ADS is copyrighted by the Addiction Research Foundation and cannot be copied without permission. In addition to the questionnaire version, a computer-administered version is available as part of the Computerized Lifestyle Assessment (Alcohol Module). Information is available from Marketing Services, Addiction Research Foundation, 33 Russell Street, Toronto, Ontario, Canada M5S 2S1, or by telephone at 416-545-6000.

Clinical Institute Withdrawal Assessment-Alcohol, Revised

Although many quantification instruments have been developed for monitoring alcohol withdrawal (Guthrie, 1989; Sellers & Naranjo, 1983; Sullivan, Sykora, Schneiderman, Naranjo, & Sellers, 1989), the best known and most extensively studied scale is the Clinical Institute Withdrawal Assessment-Alcohol (CIWA-A) and a shortened version, the CIWA-A revised (CIWA-Ar; see Table 3-1). With the CIWA-Ar, an observer rates the intensity of 10 common withdrawal symptoms, then obtains a total score that is the sum of the 10 ratings.

A study of the CIWA-Ar predicted that those with a score of >15 were at increased risk for severe alcohol withdrawal (relative risk [RR], 3.72; 95% confidence interval [CI] 2.85–4.85); the higher the score, the greater the risk. In addition to indicating severe withdrawal, high CIWA scores also are predictors of seizures and delirium (Naranjo et al., 1983; Young et al., 1987).

The CIWA has well-documented reliability, reproducibility, and validity based on comparison to ratings by expert clinicians (Knott et al., 1981; Sullivan et al., 1989; Wiehl et al., 1994). From 30 signs and symptoms, the scale has been carefully refined to a list of 10 signs and symptoms in the CIWA-Ar (Wiehl et al., 1994). It is thus easy to use and has been shown to be feasible to use in a variety of clinical settings, including detoxification units (Hoey et al., 1994; Naranjo et al., 1983), psychiatry units (Heinala, et al, 1990), and general medical/surgical wards (Katta, 1991; Young, et al, 1987).

The CIWA and CIWA-Ar can be administered by trained nonmedical personnel, such as detoxification unit workers or research assistants. The instrument also has been adapted for benzodiazepine withdrawal assessment (Clinical Institute Withdrawal Assessment-Benzodiazepine).

Drinker Inventory of Consequences

The Drinker Inventory of Consequences (DrInC) was developed to provide a comprehensive assessment of drinking problems and consequences, separate from consumption and dependence. Unlike the ASI, which assesses functional impairment across dimensions without reference to a specific causal connection to drinking, the DrInC asks the respondent to make a connection between drinking and his or her problems.

The DrInC is a paper and pencil questionnaire that can be completed in 5 to 10 minutes. It asks about physical consequences ranging from hangovers to impact on sexual functioning;

intrapersonal consequences such as guilt, shame, loss of interest, and loss of spirituality; social responsibility consequences relating to failure to meet obligations; interpersonal consequences regarding family and friends; and impulse control consequences, including motor vehicle crashes, fights, and arrests. It also contains a number of reverse-scored items as a validity check against blanket denial of all problems.

The advantage of the DrInC is that it is quick and simple to administer. The disadvantage is that, because it is a paper and pencil questionnaire, there is no opportunity for a clinician or interviewer to probe responses.

Recovery Attitude and Treatment Evaluator

The Recovery Attitude and Treatment Evaluator (RAATE-CE) was designed to quantify patient resistance and impediments to addiction treatment.

The RAATE-CE is a clinician-rated structured interview that assesses five areas relevant to substance abuse treatment planning decisions: (1) degree of resistance to treatment, (2) degree of resistance to continuing care, (3) acuity of biomedical problems, (4) acuity of psychiatric problems, and (5) extent of social, family, and/or environmental systems that are not supportive of recovery (Mee-Lee, 1988). It is designed to be administered by a trained counselor and requires approximately 35 minutes to complete.

Structured Clinical Interview for DSM-IV

The Structured Clinical Interview for DSM-IV (SCID) is a widely used, semistructured interview that obtains Axis I and II diagnoses using DSM-IV criteria. The SCID is designed for use with psychiatric, medical, or community-based normal adults (Spitzer et al., 1989). It is composed of one module for each major syndrome group in the DSM-IV: anxiety disorders, affective disorders, psychotic disorders, and substance use disorders. Each module may stand on its own for assessment of that particular diagnostic syndrome.

Each question on the SCID corresponds to a specific DSM-IV criterion. The questions are sequenced to carefully obey the decision rule process and to yield a diagnosis only if the patient meets all requisite DSM-IV criteria. Although it does measure criterion-based symptomatology, the SCID is too limited for a comprehensive treatment evaluation and should be supplemented with an instrument that has been designed for severity assessment, such as the ASI or the DrInC.

The SCID is designed for use by a clinical evaluator trained at the masters or doctoral level, although in research settings it has been used by bachelor's level technicians with extensive training. Administration of Axis I and Axis II batteries may require more than 2 hours each for patients with multiple diagnoses. The Psychoactive Substance Use Disorders module may be administered by itself in 30 to 60 minutes, depending on the extent of the patient's substance use history and current involvement.

NIAAA'S STEPS IN ASSESSMENT FOR ALCOHOL USE DISORDERS

Step 1: Assess for Alcohol Use Disorders

Determine whether there is a *maladaptive pattern of alcohol use*, causing *clinically significant impairment* or *distress*. It is important to assess the severity and extent of all alcohol-related symptoms to inform your decisions about management. The following list of symptoms is adapted from the *Diagnostic and Statistical Manual of Mental Disorders, 4th edition (DSM-IV), Revised.* Sample assessment questions are available online at *http:www.niaaa.nih.gov/guide.*

Determine whether, in the past 12 months, your patient's drinking has **repeatedly** caused or contributed to

- ☐ **risk** of bodily harm (drinking and driving, operating machinery, swimming)
- ☐ **relationship** trouble (family or friends)
- ☐ **role failure** (interference with home, work, or school obligations)
- ☐ **run-ins** with the law (arrests or other legal problems)

If yes to **one or more** ⟶ your patient has **alcohol abuse.**
In either case, proceed to assess for dependence symptoms.

Determine whether, in the past 12 months, your patient has

- ☐ **not been able to stick to drinking limits** (repeatedly gone over them)
- ☐ **not been able to cut down or stop** (repeated failed attempts)
- ☐ **shown tolerance** (needed to drink a lot more to get the same effect)
- ☐ **shown signs of withdrawal** (tremors, sweating, nausea, or insomnia when trying to quit or cut down)
- ☐ **kept drinking despite problems** (recurrent physical or psychological problems)
- ☐ **spent a lot of time drinking** (or anticipating or recovering from drinking)
- ☐ **spent less time on other matters** (activities that had been important or pleasurable)

If yes to **three or more** ⟶ your patient has **alcohol dependence.**

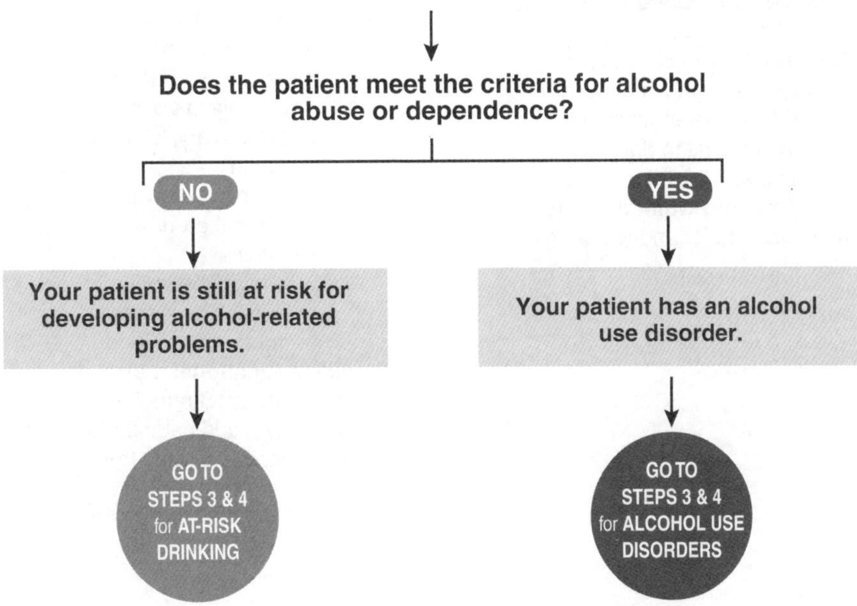

Step 2: Advise and Assist (Brief Intervention)

- **State your conclusion and recommendation clearly:**
  - "You are drinking more than is medically safe." Relate to patient's concerns and medical findings, if present. (Consider using the chart on page 25 to show increased risk.)
  - "I strongly recommend that you cut down (or quit)." (See page 29 for advice considerations)
- **Gauge readiness** to change drinking habits:
  "Are you willing to consider making changes in your drinking?"

↓

Is the patient ready to commit to change at this time?

NO

Do not be discouraged—ambivalence is common. Your advice has likely prompted a change in your patient's thinking, a positive change in itself. With continued reinforcement, your patient may decide to take action. For now,

- **Restate your concern** about his or her health.
- **Encourage reflection:** Ask patients to weigh what they like about drinking versus their reasons for cutting down. What are the major barriers to change?
- **Reaffirm your willingness to help** when he or she is ready.

YES

- **Help set a goal:** Cut down to within maximum limits (see Step 1) or abstain for a period of time.
- **Agree on a plan**, including
  - what specific steps the patient will take (e.g., not go to a bar after work, measure all drinks at home, alternate alcoholic and non-alcoholic beverages)
  - how drinking will be tracked (diary, kitchen calendar)
  - how the patient will manage high-risk situations
  - who might be willing to help, such as a spouse or nondrinking friends
- **Provide educational materials.** See page 26 for "Strategies for Cutting Down" and page 27 for other materials available from NIAAA.

Step 3: Continue Support

Document alcohol use and review goals at each visit (see the NIAAA web site for downloadable progress notes).

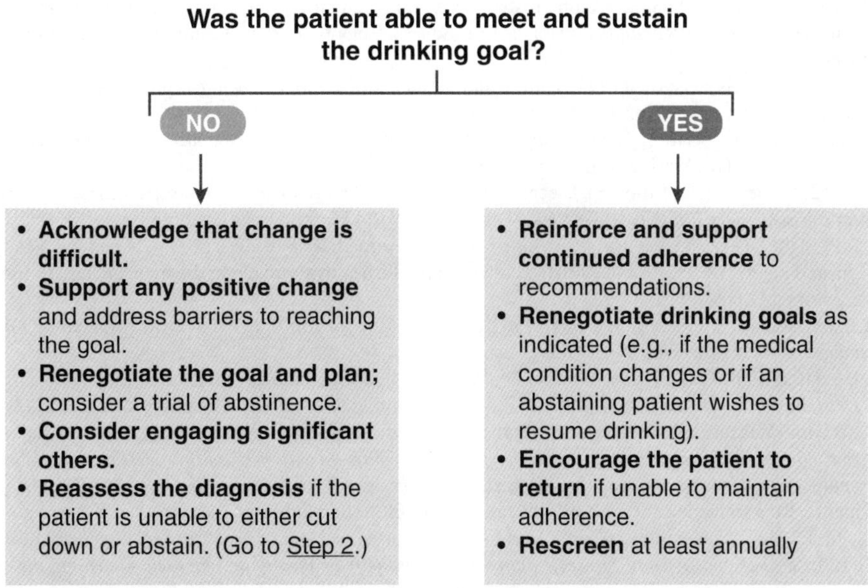

Source: Adapted from National Institute on Alcohol Abuse and Alcoholism. (2005). *Helping patients who drink too much. A clinician's* guide. NIH Publication No. 07-3769; revised January 2007. Rockville, MD: NIAAA, National Institutes of Health. Available at http://pubs.niaaa.nih.gov/publications/Practitioner/CliniciansGuide2005/clinicians_guide5_help_p.htm. Accessed September 24, 2009.

CONCLUSION

All of the assessment measures discussed, particularly when incorporated into treatment planning in some combination, can be expected to improve the uniformity, comprehensiveness, and interagency or interprovider reliability of clinical assessment. Despite the costs of training, staff adaptation, and additional time for the duration of administration, these gains can be expected to yield improvements in time and, hopefully, cost efficiency.

Source

Adapted from Gastfriend, D. R., Baker, S. L., Najavits, L. M., & Reif, S. (2003). Assessment. In A. W. Graham, T. K. Schultz, R. K. Ries, & B. B. Wilford. (Eds.). *Principles of addiction medicine.* (3rd ed.). Chevy Chase, MD: American Society of Addiction Medicine.

REFERENCES

Academic ED SBIRT Research Collaborative. (2007). The impact of screening, brief intervention, and referral for treatment on emergency department patients' alcohol use. *Annals of Emergency Medicine*, 50, 6, 699-710, 710.e1-6.

Allen, J. P., & Columbus, M. (1995). *Assessing alcohol problems: A guide for clinicians and researchers. NIAAA treatment handbook*, series 4. Rockville, MD: National Institute on Alcohol Abuse and Alcoholism.

Allen, J. P., & Litten, R. Z. (1998). Screening instruments and biochemical screening tests. In A. W. Graham, & T. K. Schultz (Eds.), *Principles of addiction medicine* (2nd ed.). Chevy Chase, MD: American Society of Addiction Medicine.

American Psychiatric Association. (1994). *Diagnostic and statistical manual of mental disorders, 4th Edition (DSM-IV)*. Washington, DC: American Psychiatric Press.

American Psychiatric Association. (2000). *Diagnostic and statistical manual of mental disorders, Fourth Edition, Text Revision (DSM-IV-TR)*. Washington, DC: American Psychiatric Press.

Babor, T. F., de la Fuente, J. R., Saunders, J., et al. (1992). AUDIT: *The alcohol use disorders identification test: Guidelines for use in primary health care.* Geneva, Switzerland: World Health Organization.

Babor, T. F., McRee, B. G., Kassebaum, P. A., Grimaldi, P. L., Ahmed, K., & Bray, J. (2007). Screening, Brief Intervention, and Referral to Treatment (SBIRT): Toward a public health approach to the management of substance abuse. *Substance Abuse*, 28, 3, 7-30.

Coups, E. J., Gaba, A., & Orleans, T. (2004). Physician screening for multiple behavioral risk factors. *American Journal of Preventive Medicine*, 27, 2S, 34-41.

Ewing, J. A. (1984). The CAGE questionnaire. *Journal of the American Medical Association*, 252, 1907.

Fiellin, D. A., Butler, R., D'Onofrio, G., Brown, R. L., & O'Connor, P. G. (2002). The physician's role in caring for patients with substance use disorders: Implications for medical education and training. In *Project mainstream: Strategic plan for interdisciplinary faculty development—Arming the nation's health professional workforce for a new approach to substance use disorders: Part II. Discipline-specific recommendations for faculty development.* Providence, RI: Association for Medical Education and Research in Substance Abuse.

Fleming, M. F. (2002). Screening, assessment, and intervention for substance use disorders in general health care settings. In *Project mainstream: Strategic plan for interdisciplinary faculty development—Arming the nation's health professional workforce for a new approach to substance use disorders, Part I. Evidence supporting the strategic plan.* Providence, RI: Association for Medical Education and Research in Substance Abuse.

Foy, A., March, S., & Drinkwater, V. (1988). Use of an objective clinical scale in the assessment and management of alcohol withdrawal in a large general hospital. *Alcoholism: Clinical and Experimental Research,* 12, 360-364.

Gastfriend, D. R., Baker, S. L., Najavits, L. M., & Reif, S. (2003). Assessment. In A. W. Graham, T. K. Schultz, R. K. Ries, & B. B. Wilford (Eds.), *Principles of addiction medicine* (3rd ed.). Chevy Chase, MD: American Society of Addiction Medicine.

Gastfriend, D. R., Filstead, W. J., Reif S., & Najavits, L. (1995). Validity of assessing treatment readiness in patients with substance use disorders. *American Journal on Addictions*, 4, 5, 254-260.

Gastfriend, D. R., & McLellan, A. T. (1997). Treatment matching: Theoretic and practical implications. *Medical Clinics of North America,* 81, 4, 1-22.

Guthrie, S. K. (1989). The treatment of alcohol withdrawal. *Pharmacotherapy*, 9, 3, 131-143.

Hasin, D. (1991). Diagnostic interviews for assessment: Background, reliability, validity. *Alcohol Health & Research World*, 15, 293-302.

Hedlund, J. L., & Vieweg, B. W. (1984). The Michigan Alcoholism Screening Test (MAST): A comprehensive review. *Journal of Operational Psychiatry*, 15, 55-64.

Heinala, P., Pieponen, T., & Heikkinen, H. (1990). Diazepam loading in alcohol withdrawal: Clinical pharmacokinetics. *International Journal of Clinical Pharmacology, Therapy and Toxicology*, 28, 211-217.

Hodgins, D., & el-Guebaly, N. (1992). More data on the Addiction Severity Index: Reliability and validity with the mentally ill substance abuser. *Journal of Nervous and Mental Disease*, 180, 197-201.

Hoey, L. L., Nahun, A., & Vance-Bryan, K. (1994). A retrospective review and assessment of benzodiazepines in the treatment of alcohol withdrawal in hospitalized patients. *Pharmacotherapy*, 14, 572-578.

Institute of Medicine. (1990). *Broadening the base of treatment for alcohol problems: A report of a study by a committee of the Institute of Medicine.* Division of Mental Health and Behavioral Medicine. Washington, DC: National Academy Press.

Isenhart, C. (1994). Motivational subtypes in an inpatient sample of substance abusers. *Addictive Behaviors*, 19, 463-475.

Kasser, C. L., Geller, A., Howell, E. F., et al. (1997). Detoxification: Principles and protocols. In *Topics in addiction medicine.* Chevy Chase, MD: American Society of Addiction Medicine.

Katta, B. B. (1991). Nifedapine for protracted withdrawal syndrome. *Canadian Journal of Psychiatry*, 36, 155.

Knott, D. H., Lerner, D., Davis-Knott, T., & Fink, R. D. (1981). Decision for alcohol detoxification: A method to standardize patient evaluation. *Postgraduate Medicine*, 69, 65-76.

Kranzler, H., Kadden, R., Babor, T., Tennen, H., & Rounsaville, B. J. (1996). Validity of the SCID in substance abuse patients. *Addiction*, 91, 859-868.

LaJeunesse, C., & Thorenson, R. (1988). Generalizing a predictor of male alcoholic treatment outcomes. *International Journal of Addiction,* 23, 183-205.

Letteri, D., Nelson, J., & Sayers, M. (1985). *Alcoholism treatment assessment research instruments.* Rockville, MD: National Institute on Alcohol Abuse and Alcoholism.

Mattson, M. E., Allen, J. P., Longabaugh R., Nickless, C. J., Connors, G. J., & Kadden, R. M. (1994). A chronological review of empirical studies matching alcoholic clients to treatment. *Journal of Studies on Alcohol*, 12(Suppl), 16-29.

McGahan, P., Griffith, J., Parente, R., et al. (1986). Composite scores from the Addiction Severity Index. Pittsburgh, PA: Penn-VA Center for Studies of Addiction (unpublished manuscript).

McLellan, A. T., Luborsky, L., & Woody, G. E. (1980). An improved diagnostic evaluation instrument for substance abuse patients: The Addiction Severity Index. *Journal of Nervous and Mental Diseases*, 168, 26-33.

McLellan, A. T., Luborsky, L., Cacciola, J., Griffith, J., Evans, F., Barr, H. L., et al. (1985). New data from the addiction severity index—Reliability and validity in three centers. *Journal of Nervous and Mental Diseases*, 173, 412-423.

McLellan, A. T., Kushner, H., Metzger, D., Peters, R., Smith, I., Grissom, G., et al. (1992). The fifth edition of the Addiction Severity Index. *Journal of Substance Abuse Treatment*, 9,199-213.

Mee-Lee, D. (1988). An instrument for treatment progress and matching: The Recovery Attitude and Treatment Evaluator (RAATE). *Journal of Substance Abuse Treatment*, 5, 183-186.

Mee-Lee, D., Shulman, G., Fishman, M., Gastfriend, D., & Griffiths, J. H. (2001). *ASAM patient placement criteria for the treatment of substance-related disorders, second edition-revised (PPC-2R).* Chevy Chase, MD: American Society of Addiction Medicine.

Mee-Lee, D., Shulman, G., & Gartner, L. (1996). *Patient placement criteria for the treatment of substance-related disorders, Second Edition (PPC-2).* Chevy Chase, MD: American Society of Addiction Medicine.

Miller, W. R., Tonigan, J. S., & Longabaugh, R. (1995). *The drinker inventory of consequences (DrInC): An instrument for assessing adverse consequences of alcohol abuse; test manual (NIAAA Project MATCH Monograph Series 4).* Washington, DC: National Institute on Alcohol Abuse and Alcoholism.

Najavits, L. M., Gastfriend, D. R., Nakayama, E. Y., Barber, J. P., Blaine, J., Frank, A., et al. (1996). A measure of readiness for substance abuse treatment: Psychometric properties of the RAATE research interview. *American Journal on Addictions*, 6, 74-82.

Naranjo, C. A., Sellers, E. M., Chater, K., Iversen, P., Roach, C., & Sykora, K. (1983). Nonpharmacologic intervention with acute alcohol withdrawal. *Clinical Pharmacology and Therapeutics*, 34, 214-219.

National Institute on Alcohol Abuse and Alcoholism. (NIAAA) (2005). *Helping patients who drink too much. A clinician's guide.* NIH Publication No. 07-3769; revised January 2007. Rockville, MD: NIAAA, National Institutes of Health.

Prochaska, J. O., & DiClemente, C. C. (1992). Stages of change in the modification of problem behaviors. *Progress in Behavior Modification*, 28, 183-218.

Robins, L. N., Helzer, J. E., Croughan, J., & Ratcliff, K. S. (1981). National Institute of Mental Health Diagnostic Interview Schedule. *Archives of General Psychiatry*, 38, 4, 381-389.

Sellers, E. M., & Naranjo, C. A. (1983). New strategies for the treatment of alcohol withdrawal. *Psychopharmacology Bulletin*, 22, 88-91.

Selzer, M. L. (1971). The Michigan Alcoholism Screening Test: The quest for a new diagnostic instrument. *American Journal of Psychiatry*, 127, 1653-1658.

Skinner, H. A., & Allen, B. A. (1982). Alcohol dependence syndrome: Measurement and validation. *Journal of Abnormal Psychology,* 91, 199-209.

Skinner, H. A., & Horn, J. L. (1984). *Alcohol dependence scale: Users guide.* Toronto, Ontario: Addiction Research Foundation.

Skre, I., Onstad, S., Torgersen, S., & Kringlen, E. (1991). High interrater reliability for the Structured Clinical Interview for DSM-IIIR Axis I. *Acta Psychiatrica Scandinavica*, 84, 167-173.

Smith, B., Hoffman, N., & Nederhoed, R. (1992). The development and reliability of the RAATE-CE. *Journal of Substance Abuse*, 4, 355-363.

Spitzer, R. L., Williams, J. B., Mirian, G., et al. (1989). *Instruction manual for the structured interview for DSM-IIIR.* New York: Biometrics Research Dept., New York State Psychiatric Institute, May 1.

Spitzer, R. L., Williams, J. B., Gibbon, M., & First, M. B. (1992). The Structured Clinical Interview for DSM-IIIR (SCID) I: History, rationale and description. *Archives of General Psychiatry*, 49, 624-629.

Sullivan, J. T., Sykora K., Schneiderman J., Naranjo, C. A., & Sellers, E. M. (1989). Assessment of alcohol withdrawal: The revised clinical institute withdrawal assessment for alcohol scale (CIWA-Ar). *British Journal of the Addictions*, 84, 1353-1357.

Young, G. P., Rores, C., Murphy, C., & Dailey, R. H. (1987). Intravenous phenobarbital for alcohol withdrawal and convulsions. *Annals of Emergency Medicine*, 16, 847-850.

Wiehl, W.O., Hayner, G., & Galloway, G. (1994). Haight Ashbury Free Clinics drug detoxification protocols, Part 4: Alcohol. *Journal of Psychoactive Drugs*, 26, 57-59.

Williams, J. B., Gibbon, M., First, M. B., Spitzer, R. L., Davies, M., Borus, J., et al. (1992). The Structured Clinical Interview for DSM-IIIR (SCID), II. Multisite test-retest reliability. *Archives of General Psychiatry*, 49, 630-636.

APPENDIX B

Selected Nonpharmacologic Therapies for Alcohol Use Disorders

Experts recommend that some form of psychosocial therapy should be considered as a treatment option for all patients who seek help for a substance use disorder (Rounsaville & Carroll, 2003). Many treatment programs use psychosocial approaches to help patients acquire the skills necessary to avoid a relapse after they achieve initial abstinence. The objective of such therapies is to change the patient's behavior regarding alcohol consumption.

Psychosocial approaches include behavioral therapy, cognitive therapy, various types of psychotherapy, counseling, and other rehabilitative strategies. Although they do not constitute formal treatment, Alcoholics Anonymous and other self- and mutual-help programs provide important supports for recovery and often are included in this category.

MOTIVATIONAL ENHANCEMENT THERAPY

Motivational enhancement therapy (MET) is a client-centered counseling approach that has been used successfully with alcoholics and with individuals with other substance use disorders (Stephens, Roffman, & Simpson, 1994). Its purpose is to initiate behavior change by helping patients resolve ambivalence about engaging in treatment and stopping their alcohol or drug use. Many patients with alcohol dependence are in early stages of change (e.g., the precontemplation stage) at the time they enter treatment and do not think they have a problem with alcohol.

MET employs strategies to evoke internally generated change in a patient, by highlighting discrepancies between the patient's own goals and his or her behaviors (in particular *drinking* behaviors), and providing structured feedback to stimulate the patient's motivation to change (DiClemente, Bellino, & Neavins, 1999; Miller, 1996).

MET initially focuses on providing feedback generated from the assessment to stimulate discussion regarding personal substance use and to elicit self-motivational statements. Motivational interviewing principles are used to strengthen motivation and build a plan for change. Coping strategies for high-risk situations are suggested and discussed (Miller, 1996).

The therapist monitors change, reviews the strategies being used by the patient, and continues to encourage commitment to change or sustained abstinence. MET, which is based on the principles of motivational psychology, does not prescribe to the patient a step-by-step process through recovery but strives to motivate the individual to use his or her own resources to change behavior. Additional principles of MET include avoiding confrontation, rolling with resistance and promoting self-efficacy.

COGNITIVE-BEHAVIORAL THERAPY

Cognitive-behavioral therapy (CBT) is among the most well-studied and empirically supported treatments for addiction. CBT strategies are anchored in the theory that learning processes play a critical role in the development of maladaptive behavior patterns (National Institute on Drug Abuse [NIDA], 2000). In formal CBT, patients practice behavioral or cognitive skills to identify and correct problematic behaviors, and cope with high-risk situations through rehearsal, role playing, and homework. Variations of CBT are widely used in alcoholism treatment under the label of "relapse prevention."

Specifically, CBT focuses on identifying and changing thoughts and behaviors that contribute to compulsive alcohol use and/or place the individual at high risk of relapsing. CBT helps patients identify triggers for use, such as people (e.g., drinking friends, irritating coworkers), places (particular bars, clubs, or restaurants), or emotions (sadness or anger).

The relapse prevention approach consists of a collection of strategies intended to enhance self-control. For example, through modeling and role playing, CBT teaches patients effective drink-refusal skills. Patients are taught to avoid high-risk situations or triggers whenever they can, and to cope effectively with situations or triggers that are unavoidable. Specific techniques include exploring the positive and negative consequences of continued use (sometimes referred to as "functional analysis"); self-monitoring to facilitate early recognition of cravings and high-risk situations; and developing strategies for coping with and avoiding high-risk situations and the desire to use. A central element of this treatment is anticipating the problems patients are likely to meet and helping them develop effective coping strategies (Marlatt & Gordon, 1985).

CBT encourages the drinker to pursue activities incompatible with drinking and to identify and cope with negative thinking (McCrady, 1994). Research indicates that the skills individuals learn through relapse prevention therapy remain after the completion of treatment. Various studies have evaluated the efficacy of CBT (Longabaugh & Morgenstern, 1999; Project MATCH Research Group, 1997). In one study, most patients who received this CBT approach maintained the gains they made in treatment throughout the following year (Marlatt & Gordon, 1985).

INDIVIDUAL COUNSELING

Counseling focuses directly on reducing or stopping the addicted individual's use of alcohol and other drugs. It also addresses related areas of impaired functioning, such as employment status, illegal activity, and family/social relations, as well as the content and structure of the patient's recovery program. Through its emphasis on short-term behavioral goals, counseling helps the patient develop coping strategies and tools for abstaining from alcohol use and then maintaining that abstinence (McLellan, Arndt, Metzger, Woody, & O'Brien, 1993).

Most addiction counselors encourage participation in Twelve Step or other mutual support programs and make referrals for needed medical, psychiatric, employment, and other services. Individual counseling may be employed at all levels of care—in Level I treatment, for example, patients are often encouraged to attend counseling sessions one or two times per week (McLellan, Woody, Luborsky, & O'Brien, 1988).

GROUP THERAPIES

Group therapies are widely used in the treatment of substance use disorders to address issues such as initiating abstinence and engaging the patient in a recovery process, relapse prevention (Daley & Marlatt, 1997), anger management (Reilly & Shropshire, 2000), and co-occurring psychiatric disorders (Khantzian, Golden, & McAuliffe, 1999).

Treatment groups provide a context in which addicted persons can gain support, encouragement, feedback, and confrontation from peers who understand from personal experience how addicted individuals think, feel, and act, including the manipulations, schemes, and diversions they sometimes use to rationalize their substance use and other maladaptive behaviors. Specific strategies include (1) providing education on addiction, recovery, and relapse; (2) resolving ambivalence by overcoming denial and enhancing motivation to change; (3) instilling hope and optimism for change; (4) providing an opportunity to give and receive feedback, support, and/or confrontation from peers; (5) teaching recovery skills to manage the addictive disorder over the long term; (6) understanding and resolving problems contributing to or resulting from the addictive disorder, rather than avoiding such problems; (7) providing a context in which the patient can identify with others and give and receive support; (8) creating an experience of positive membership in a recovery-oriented group in which feelings, thoughts, and conflicts can be freely expressed; (9) preparing the patient for involvement in long-term treatment; and (10) facilitating the patient's interest in participating in self-help programs in addition to treatment groups (Daley, Mercer, & Carpenter, 1998; Washton, 1997). One of the advantages cited for the group modality is the sense of credibility and mutual collaboration that may be attributed to peers who "have been there" as opposed to professionals who may or may not speak from personal experience.

TWELVE STEP PROGRAMS

Alcoholics Anonymous (AA) and similar self-help groups outline 12 consecutive activities, or steps, that individuals should achieve during the recovery process. For example, these steps specify that drinkers must admit that they are powerless over alcohol, make a moral inventory of themselves, admit the nature of their wrongs, make a list of everyone they have harmed, and make amends to those people. One of the strengths of Twelve Step methods is an emphasis on spirituality and personal growth.

Many individuals become involved with AA before entering professional treatment. Others engage as part of their professional treatment, as aftercare following professional treatment, or in place of professional treatment.

Most treatment programs encourage patients to attend regular meetings of AA or similar self-help groups that are based on a Twelve Step philosophy (Fuller & Hiller-Sturmhöfel, 2003).

TWELVE STEP FACILITATION

Twelve Step facilitation (TSF) is a formal treatment approach designed to introduce patients to and involve them in AA and similar Twelve Step programs. TSF guides individuals through the first five steps of the AA program and promotes AA affiliation and involvement. For example, therapists who use TSF actively encourage their patients to attend AA meetings, maintain a journal of their AA attendance and participation, obtain a sponsor, and work on completing the first five steps. Participants also receive reading assignments from the AA literature.

BRIEF INTERVENTION

Many persons with alcohol-related problems do not seek the help of an alcoholism treatment specialist, but rather receive care from a primary care physician. Brief Intervention therapies are ideally suited to such settings. Such treatments can be completed in four or five office visits (Wilford, 2008). Brief intervention may also take advantage of a "teachable moment" in an emergency department, in the context of medical treatment for an alcohol-related illness or injury. Brief Intervention is typically useful for low to medium severity cases. It should be embedded in a full continuum of Screening, Brief Intervention, Referral, and Treatment (SBIRT). The availability and use of referral and more comprehensive specialty treatment is essential for the management of more severe cases, and those cases that are not amenable to Brief Intervention.

In general, Brief Intervention begins with an assessment of the extent of the patient's alcohol-related problems (e.g., impaired liver function or alcohol-related problems at work) and a discussion of the potential health consequences of continued drinking. The health care professional then offers advice on strategies to cut down on drinking (for non–alcohol-dependent patients only) or to abstain from drinking (for both dependent and nondependent patients). Such strategies can include setting specific goals for reducing the number of drinks consumed per day or per week and agreeing to written contracts that specify measures of progress toward changes in drinking behavior (Fuller & Hiller-Sturmhöfel, 2003).

COMMUNITY REINFORCEMENT APPROACH

The Community Reinforcement Approach (CRA) initially was used in the treatment of cocaine addiction, but has been adapted to other substances including alcohol. The treatment goal is to sustain abstinence through learning new life skills that will help sustain abstinence. Patients become connected to aspects of community life without substance use, and abstinence is reinforced by their newfound successes. Patients typically attend counseling sessions where they focus on improving family relations, learn a variety of skills to minimize their substance use, receive vocational counseling, and develop new recreational activities and social networks.

FAMILY AND COUPLES THERAPY

The effects of alcohol dependence are far reaching and patients' family members and loved ones also are affected by the disorder. By including family members and partners in the treatment process, education about factors that are important to the patient's recovery (such as establishing a substance-free environment) can be conveyed. Family members and partners can provide social support to the patient and can help motivate them to remain in treatment.

Research has demonstrated the effectiveness of behavioral couples therapy (BCT) in decreasing alcohol consumption, and enhancing marital satisfaction (Fals-Stewart, 2000). Studies have also shown that adding BCT to disulfiram treatment can augment treatment.

ASSERTIVE COMMUNITY TREATMENT (ACT)

Assertive Community Treatment (ACT) involves active outreach to persons who need a support system that facilitates living and functioning adequately in the community. ACT encompasses comprehensive services designed to engage and retain patients in treatment and assist them in managing daily living, obtaining work, building and strengthening family and friendship networks, managing symptoms and crises, and preventing relapse.

CASE MANAGEMENT

Case management is a collaborative process that involves assessment, planning, implementation, coordination, monitoring, and evaluation of options and services to meet an individual's health needs, using available resources. It focuses on promoting quality and cost effective outcomes (Definition of the National Case Management Task Force; National Commission for Certifying Agencies, 1993).

REFERENCES

Agency for Health Care Policy and Research. (1999). *Pharmacotherapy for alcohol dependence* [Summary, Evidence Report/Technology Assessment Number 3]. Rockville, MD: AHRQ, U.S. Department of Health and Human Services. Available at http://www.ahrq.gov/clinic/epcsums/alcosumm.htm. Accessed September 25, 2009.

Anton, R. F., O'Malley, S. S., Ciraulo, D. A., Cisler, R. A., Couper, D., Donovan, D. M., et al. (2006). Combined pharmacotherapies and behavioral interventions for alcohol dependence – The COMBINE Study: A randomized controlled trial. *Journal of the American Medical Association*, 295, 17, 2003-2017.

Brown, S. A., & Schuckit, M. A. (1988). Changes in depression among abstinent alcoholics. *Journal of Studies on Alcohol*, 49, 412-417.

Carroll, K. M., & Schottenfeld, R. (1997). Nonpharmacologic approaches to substance abuse treatment. *The Medical Clinics of North America, 81,* 4, 927-944.

Crits-Christoph, P. L., Siqueland, L., Blaine J., Frank, A., Luborsky, L., Onken, L. S., et al. (1999). Psychosocial treatments for cocaine dependence: National Institute on Drug Abuse Collaborative Cocaine Treatment Study. *Archives of General Psychiatry*, 56, 493-502.

Daley, D. C., & Marlatt, G. A. (1997). *Managing your drug or alcohol problem: Therapist guide.* San Antonio, TX: The Psychological Corporation.

Daley, D. C., Marlatt, G. A., & Spotts, C. E. (2003). Relapse prevention: Clinical models and intervention strategies. In A. W. Graham, T. K. Schultz, M. F. Mayo-Smith, R. K. Ries, & B. B. Wilford (Eds.), *Principles of addiction medicine (3rd ed.).* Chevy Chase, MD: American Society of Addiction Medicine.

Daley, D. C., Mercer, D., & Carpenter, G. (1998). *Group drug counseling manual.* Holmes Beach, FL: Learning Publications, Inc.

Daley, D. C., & Roth, L. (2001). *When symptoms return: A guide to relapse in psychiatric* illness (2nd ed.). Holmes Beach, FL: Learning Publications.

Delaney, H. D., Forcehimes, A. A., Campbell, W. P., & Smith, B. W. (2009). Integrating spirituality into alcohol treatment. *Journal of Clinical Psychology*, 65, 2, 185-198.

DiClemente, C., Bellino, L., & Neavins, T. (1999).Motivation for change and alcoholism treatment. *Alcohol Research & Health*, 23, 2, 78-85.

Dimeff, L. A., & Marlatt, G. A. (1995). Relapse prevention. In R. Hester, & W. Miller (Eds.), *Handbook of alcoholism treatment approaches* (2nd ed., pp. 176-194). Boston: Allyn & Bacon.

Doering, P. L. (1999). Substance-related disorders: Alcohol, nicotine, and caffeine. In J. T. DiPiro, R. L. Talbert, G. C. Yee et al. (Eds.), *Pharmacotherapy: A pathophysiologic approach* (4th ed.). Stamford, CT: Appleton & Lange.

Dongier, M. (2005). Psychopharmacology for the clinician. *Reviews of Psychiatry and Neuroscience (Canada), 30,* 3.

Donovan, D. M., Anton, R. F., Miller, W. R., Longabaugh, R., Hosking, J. D., & Youngblood, M. (2008). Combined pharmacotherapies and behavioral interventions for alcohol dependence (The COMBINE Study): Examination of posttreatment drinking outcomes. *Journal of Studies on Alcohol and Drugs*, 69, 1, 5-13.

Dundon, W. D., Pettinati, H. M., Lynch, K. G., Xie, H., Varillo, K. M., Makadon, C., et al. (2008). The therapeutic alliance in medical-based interventions impacts outcome in treating alcohol dependence. *Drug and Alcohol Dependence, 95,* 3, 230-236.

Ernst, D. B., Pettinati, H. M., Weiss, R. D., Donovan, D. M., & Longabaugh, R. (2008). An intervention for treating alcohol dependence: Relating elements of Medical Management to patient outcomes with implications for primary care. *Annals of Family Medicine, 6,* 5, 435-440.

Fals-Stewart, W., O'Farrell, T. J., Feehan, M., Birchler, G. R., Tiller, S., & McFarlin, S. K. (2000). Behavioral couples therapy versus individual-based treatment for male substance-abusing patients. An evaluation of significant individual change and comparison of improvement rates. *J Subst Abuse Treat, 18,* 3, 249-254.

Finney, J. W., & Moos, R. H. (2003). Effects of setting, duration, and amount on treatment outcomes. In A. W. Graham, T. K. Schultz, M. F. Mayo-Smith, R. K. Ries, & B. B. Wilford (Eds.) *Principles of addiction medicine* (3rd ed.). Chevy Chase, MD: American Society of Addiction Medicine.

Fuller, R. K., & Hiller-Sturmhöfel (2003). PRIVATE The treatment of alcoholism: A review. In A. W. Graham, T. K. Schultz, M. F. Mayo-Smith, R. K. Ries, & B. B. Wilford (Eds.), *Principles of addiction medicine* (3rd ed.). Chevy Chase, MD: American Society of Addiction Medicine.

Galanter, M, (2008). The concept of spirituality in relation to addiction recovery and general psychiatry. *Recent Developments in Alcoholism, 18,* 125-40.

Gastfriend, D. R., Garbutt, J. C., Pettinati, H. M., & Forman, R. F. (2007). Reduction in heavy drinking as a treatment outcome in alcohol dependence. *Journal of Substances Abuse Treatment, 33,* 1, 71-80.

Gottheil, E., Thornton, C., & Weinstein, S. (2002). Effectiveness of high versus low structure individual counseling for substance abuse. *The American Journal on Addiction, 11,* 4, 279-290.

Grant, B. F., & Harford, T. C. (1995). Comorbidity between DSM-IV alcohol use disorders and major depression: Results of a national survey. *Drug and Alcohol Dependence, 39,*197-206.

Hesselbrock, M. N., Meyer, R. E., & Keener, J. J. (1985). Psychopathology in hospitalized alcoholics. *Archives of General Psychiatry*, 42, 1050-1055.

Hillemacher, T., & Bleich, S. (2008). Neurobiology and treatment in alcoholism – Recent findings regarding Lesch's typology of alcohol dependence. *Alcohol & Alcoholism, 43,* 3, 341-346.

Kelly, J. F., & McCrady, B. S. (2008). Twelve-step facilitation in non-specialty settings. *Recent Developments in Alcoholism, 18,* 321-346.

Kessler, R. C., Crum, R. M., Warner, L. A., Nelson, C. B., Schulenberg, J., & Anthony, J. C. (1997). Lifetime co-occurrence of DSM-IIIR alcohol abuse and dependence with other psychiatric disorders in the National Comorbidity Study. *Archives of General Psychiatry, 54,* 313-321.

Kessler, R. C., McGonagle, K. A., Zhao, S., Nelson, C. B., Hughes, M., Eshleman, S., et al. (1994). Lifetime and 12-month prevalence of DSM-IIIR psychiatric disorders in the United States. *Archives of General Psychiatry, 51,* 8-19.

Khantzian, E. J., Golden, S. J., & McAuliffe, W. E. (1999).Group therapy. In M. Galanter & H. D. Kleber (Eds.) *Textbook of substance abuse treatment* (pp. 367-378). Washington, DC: American Psychiatric Press.

Koob, G. F., Roberts, A. J., Schulteis, G., Parsons, L. H., Heyser, C. J., Hyytia, P., et al. (1998). Neurocircuitry targets in ethanol reward and dependence. *Alcoholism, Clinical and Experimental Research, 22,* 3-9.

Kranzler, H. R., & Rounsaville B. J. (1998). *Dual diagnosis: Substance abuse and comorbid medical and psychiatric disorders.* New York: Marcel Dekker.

LeMarquand, D., Pihl, R. O., & Benkelfat, C. (1994a). Serotonin and alcohol intake, abuse, and dependence: Findings of animal studies. *Biological Psychiatry, 36,* 395-421.

LeMarquand, D., Pihl, R. O., & Benkelfat, C. (1994b). Serotonin and alcohol intake, abuse, and dependence: Clinical evidence. *Biological Psychiatry, 36,* 326-337.

Longabaugh, R., & Morgenstern, J. (1999).Cognitive-behavioral coping-skills therapy for alcohol dependence. *Alcohol Research & Health, 23,* 2, 78-85.

Luborsky, L. (1984). *Principles of psychoanalytic psychotherapy: A manual for supportive-expressive (SE) treatment.* New York: Basic Books.

Maisto, S. A., Clifford, P. R., Stout, R. L., & Davis, C. M. (2008). Factors mediating the association between drinking in the first year after alcohol treatment and drinking at three years. *Journal of Studies on Alcohol and Drugs, 69,* 5, 728-737.

Marlatt, G., & Gordon, J. R. (1985). *Relapse prevention: Maintenance strategies in the treatment of addictive behaviors.* New York: Guilford Press.

Mattson, M. E., & Litten, R. Z. (2005). Combining treatments for alcoholism: Why and how? *Journal of Studies on Alcohol, 15,* 8-16.

McCrady, B. S. (1994). Alcoholics Anonymous and behavior therapy: Can habits be treated as diseases? Can diseases be treated as habits? *Journal of Consulting and Clinical Psychology*, 62, 1159?1166.

McLellan, A. T., Arndt, I., Metzger, D. S., Woody, G. E., & O'Brien, C. P. (1993). The effects of psychosocial services in substance abuse treatment. *Journal of the American Medical Association, 269,* 15, 1953-1959.

McLellan, A. T., Woody, G. E., Luborsky, L., & O'Brien, C. P. (1988). Is the counselor an "active ingredient" in substance abuse treatment? *Journal of Nervous and Mental Disease, 176,* 423-430.

Miller, W. R. (1996). Motivational interviewing: Research, practice and puzzles. *Addictive Behaviors, 61,* 6, 835-842.

Monahan, S. C., & Finney, J. W. (1996).Explaining abstinence rates following treatment for alcohol abuse: A quantitative synthesis of patient, research design, and treatment effects. *Addiction, 91,* 787–805.

Myrick, H., Anton, R. F., Li, X., Henderson, S., Drobes, D., Voronin, K., et al. (2004). Differential brain activity in alcoholics and social drinkers to alcohol cues: Relationship to craving. *Neuropsychopharmacology, 29,* 393-402.

Nace, C. P., Saxon, J. J., & Shore, N. (1983). A comparison of borderline and nonborderline alcoholic patients. *Archives of General Psychiatry, 40,* 54-56.

Najavits, L. M., Weiss, R. D., & Liese, B. S. (1995).Group cognitive-behavioral therapy for women with PTSD and Substance use disorder. *Journal of Substance Abuse Treatment, 13,* 1, 13-22.

National Commission for Certifying Agencies. (1993). *CCM certification guide.* Rolling Meadows, IL: Author.

National Institute on Alcohol Abuse and Alcoholism (NIAAA). (2008). *Helping patients who drink too much: A clinician's guide.* Bethesda, MD: NIAAA, National Institutes of Health. Available at http://www.niaaa.nih.gov/Publications/EducationTrainingMaterials/guide.htm.

National Institute on Drug Abuse (NIDA). (1993). *Cue extinction techniques* (NIDA Technology Transfer Package). Rockville, MD: NIDA, National Institutes of Health.

National Institute on Drug Abuse (NIDA). (2000). *Principles of drug addiction treatment: A research-based guide.* NIH Publication No. 00-4180. Rockville, MD: NIDA, National Institutes of Health.

Neto, D., Lambaz, R., Aguiar, P., & Chick, J. (2008). Effectiveness of sequential combined treatment in comparison with treatment as usual in preventing relapse in alcohol dependence. *Alcohol & Alcoholism, 43,* 6, 661-668.

Nunes, E. V., & Levin, F. R. (2004). Treatment of depression in patients with alcohol and other drug dependence: a meta-analysis. *Journal of the American Medical Association, 291,* 1887-1896.

Pagano, M. E., Zemore, S. E., Onder, C. C., & Stout, R. L. (2009). Predictors of initial AA-related helping: Findings from Project MATCH. *Journal of Studies on Alcohol and Drugs, 70,* 1, 117-25.

Pettinati, H. M., & Rabinowitz, A. R. (2005). Recent advances in the treatment of alcoholism. *Clinical Neuroscience Research, 5,* 151-159.

Project MATCH Research Group. (1997). Matching alcoholism treatments to client heterogeneity: Project MATCH post-treatment drinking outcomes. *Journal of Studies on Alcohol, 58,* 7-29.

Regier, D. A., Farmer, M. E., Rae, D. S., Locke, B. Z., Keith, S. J., Judd, L. L., et al. (1990). Comorbidity of mental disorders with alcohol and other drug abuse. Results from the Epidemiologic Catchment Area (ECA) Study. *Journal of the American Medical Association, 264,* 2511-2518.

Reilly, P. M., & Shropshire, M. S. (2000).Anger management group treatment for cocaine dependence: Preliminary outcomes. *American Journal of Drug and Alcohol Abuse, 26,* 2, 161-177.

Rounsaville, B. J., & Carroll, K. M. (2003). Individual psychotherapy. In A. W. Graham, T. K. Schultz, M. F. Mayo-Smith, R. K. Ries, & B. B. Wilford (Eds.), *Principles of Addiction Medicine, Third Edition.* Chevy Chase, MD: American Society of Addiction Medicine.

Schuckit, M. A. (2009). An overview of genetic influences in alcoholism. *Journal on Substance Abuse Treatment, 36,* 1, S5-14.

Stephens, R. S., Roffman, R. A., & Simpson, E. E. (1994). Treatment adult marijuana dependence: A test of the relapse prevention model. *Journal of Consulting and Clinical Psychology, 62,* 1, 92-99.

Stitzer, M., & Petry, N. (2006). Contingency management for treatment of substance abuse. *Annual Review of Clinica Psychology, 2,* 411-434.

Swift, R. (2007). Emerging approaches to managing alcohol dependence. *American Journal Health-System Pharmacy, 64*(5 Suppl 3), S12-22.

Tims, F., & Leukefeld, C. (1987). *Relapse and recovery in drug abuse.* NIDA Research Monograph 72. Rockville, MD: NIDA, National Institutes of Health.

Volkow, N. D., & Li, T. K. (2005). Drugs and alcohol: Treating and preventing abuse, addiction and their medical consequences. *Pharmacologic Therapies, 108,* 1, 3-17.

Volpicelli, J. R., Pettinati, H. M., McLellan, A. T., et al. (2001). *Combining medication and psychosocial treatments for addiction—The Brenda Approach.* New York: Guilford.

Washton, A. M. (1997). Structured outpatient group treatment. In J. H. Lowinson, P. Ruiz, R. B. Millman, & J. G. Langrod (Eds.), *Substance abuse: A comprehensive textbook* (3rd ed., pp. 440-447). Baltimore, MD: Williams & Wilkins.

Welte, J., Hynes, G., Sokolow, L., & Lyons, J. P. (1981). Effect of length of stay in inpatient alcoholism treatment on outcome. *Journal of Studies on Alcohol, 42,* 483–491.

Wilford, B. B. (2008). Screening and brief intervention: A summary of the current literature. Washington, DC: Office of National Drug Control Policy, Executive Office of the President, The White House (accessed at www.whitehousedrugpolicy.gov).

Woody, G. E., McLellan, A. T., Luborsky, L., & O'Brien, C. P. (1995). Psychotherapy in community methadone programs: A validation study. *American Journal of Psychiatry, 152,* 9, 1302-1308.

Woody, G. E., McLellan, A. T., Luborsky, L., & O'Brien, C. P. (1987). Twelve month follow-up of psychotherapy for opiate dependence. *American Journal of Psychiatry, 144,* 590-596.

APPENDIX C

Glossary of Terms

In an effort to resolve disagreements and confusion in the addiction field over the use and meaning of terms, the American Society of Addiction Medicine (ASAM) formed a Committee on Nomenclature in 1990 to select terms it believed were important to the practice of addiction medicine and to come to agreement on how those terms should be defined.

Earlier, the American Medical Association (AMA), through a Delphi process, had produced a list of 50 terms that were adjudged by a representative group of respondents to be most significant, as then currently used by the field (Rinaldi, Steindler, Wilford, & Goodwin, 1988). The most agreed-upon definition also was determined for each of the terms.

Working primarily with the AMA list but also selecting terms from their own experience as addiction specialists, members of the ASAM Committee compiled a list of 32 high priority terms and established a definition for each. The terms and definitions then were approved by the ASAM Board of Directors as recommended terminology for use in all ASAM scientific publications and for dissemination to the field.

The Committee and Board also endorsed the definition of "alcoholism" that had been developed by a special joint committee of ASAM and the National Council on Alcoholism and Drug Dependence (Morse & Flavin, 1992).

In 2008, the role of the Nomenclature Committee was assumed by ASAM's new Descriptive and Diagnostic Terminology Action Group, which was tasked by the Board of Directors with developing a nomenclature for addiction medicine that reflects current scientific knowledge and evidence-based clinical practices. Such a nomenclature has the potential to affect reimbursement practices, public policies, and public understanding of the disease of addiction.

A glossary of terms used in the ASAM *PPC-2R* is given here to help the reader interpret the criteria. *Note: An asterisk denotes a definition that has been formally adopted by ASAM's Board of Directors.*

*__Abstinence.__ Non-use of a specific substance. In recovery, non-use of any addictive psychoactive substance. May also denote cessation of an addictive behavior, such as gambling, over-eating, etc.

Abuse. The definition of "abuse" varies widely, depending on the context in which it is used and who is supplying the definition. For example, the American Psychiatric Association in its *Diagnostic and*

Statistical Manual of Mental Disorders, Fourth Edition, Text Revision (2000) defines abuse as "a maladaptive pattern of substance use, leading to clinically significant impairment or distress, as manifested by one or more behaviors."

More recently, ASAM defined abuse as use of a substance in a manner that "deviates from approved medical, legal, and social standards, generally to achieve a euphoric state ('high') or sustain an established dependence." This document employs the ASAM definition, which reflects a consensus among addiction experts.

***Addiction.** Addiction is defined by ASAM, the American Pain Society (APS), and the American Academy of Pain Medicine (AAPM) as "a primary, chronic, neurobiologic disease, with genetic, psychosocial, and environmental factors influencing its development and manifestations. It is characterized by behaviors that include one or more of the following: impaired control over drug use, compulsive use, continued use despite harm, and craving" (AAPM, APS, and ASAM, 2001).

***Addictionist.** Also, "addictionologist" or "addiction medicine specialist." A physician who specializes in addiction medicine (usually, someone certified by ASAM in addiction medicine or the American Board of Psychiatry and Neurology [ABPN] in addiction psychiatry).

Addiction-Only Services (AOS). Services directly solely at the treatment of addictive disorders. Such services are not directed at co-occurring mental disorders; for example, an AOS program typically would not accept an individual who needs psychotropic medications, and mental health issues generally would not be addressed in treatment planning or content.

Adherence/Compliance. Adherence is a term that the health care field has been increasingly using to replace the term "compliance." Both terms have been used, sometimes interchangeably, to refer to how closely patients cooperate with, follow, and take personal responsibility for the implementation of their treatment plan. The terms are often used with the more narrow sense of how well patients accomplish the goal of persistently taking medications, but also refer more broadly to all components of treatment. Assessment of patients' efforts to accomplish the goals of a treatment plan is essential to treatment success. These efforts occur along a complex spectrum from independent proactive commitment, to mentored collaboration, to passive cooperation, to reluctant partial agreement, to active resistance, to full refusal. Attempts to understand factors that promote or inhibit adherence/compliance must take into account behaviors, attitudes, willingness, and varying degrees of capacity and autonomy. "To adhere" is "to cling, cleave (to be steadfast, hold fast), to stick fast" (*Webster's Dictionary*). The term "adherence" emphasizes the patient's collaboration and participation in treatment. It contributes to a greater focus on motivational enhancement approaches that engage and empower patients. "To comply" is "to act in accordance with another's wishes, or with rules and regulations" (*Webster's Dictionary*). The term "compliance" is falling into disuse because patient engagement and responsibility to change is a goal beyond passive compliance. For further discussion see Chapter 1 (Zweben et al., 2008).

Admission. That point in an individual's relationship with an organized treatment service when the intake process has been completed and the individual is entitled to receive the services of the treatment program.

Adolescent. As used in the *PPC-2R*, an individual aged 13 through 18. The term also frequently is used to describe young adults 18 through 21 years of age, who may be more appropriately treated with adolescent services than adult services. Moreover, many states legally classify individuals as adolescents up to age 21.

***Alcoholics Anonymous.** Many individuals with alcohol dependence find help and support through AA and similar mutual help programs. AA is a national, peer-based fellowship led by nonprofessionals and is free of charge. It is structured around 12 steps that focus on acceptance of the disease of addiction and loss of control over it, surrender to a greater power, a better understanding of the negative consequences of use and how it affects others, and fellowship. "The only requirement for membership is a desire to stop drinking" (from the *Alcoholics Anonymous Preamble*).

Alcoholism. A general but not diagnostic term, typically used to describe alcohol dependence, but sometimes used more broadly to describe a variety of problems related to the use of beverage alcohol.

Ambivalence. Ambivalence is a state of mind in which an individual has concurrent but conflicting feelings about something. The person may be ambivalent about engaging in certain behavior (eating, drinking, smoking, gambling, etc.) or resisting it.

Ambulatory Detoxification. Medically monitored detoxification that that does not require admission to an inpatient, medically or clinically monitored or managed setting.

Assertive Community Treatment (ACT). ACT involves active outreach to persons who need a support system that facilitates living and functioning adequately in the community. ACT encompasses comprehensive services designed to engage and retain patients in treatment and assist them in managing daily living, obtaining work, building and strengthening family and friendship networks, managing symptoms and crises, and preventing relapse.

Assessment. Those procedures by which a program evaluates an individual's strengths, weaknesses, problems, and needs, and determines priorities so that a treatment plan can be developed.

Biomedical. Biologic and physiologic aspects of a patient's condition and thus of the assessment and treatment of the patient. In addiction treatment, biomedical problems may be the direct result of a substance use disorder or be independent of and interactive with them, thus affecting the total treatment plan and prognosis.

***Blackout.** Acute anterograde amnesia with no formation of long-term memory, resulting from the ingestion of alcohol or other drugs; that is, a period of memory loss for which there is no recall of activities.

Bundling. An approach to treatment that ties or "bundles" several treatment services together, often delivering them in a specific treatment setting. Because this approach often overlooks a patient's individual needs and can lead to inappropriate and unnecessary services, the current trend is toward "unbundled" services.

Case Management. Case management is a collaborative process which assesses, plans, implements, coordinates, monitors, and evaluates the options and services to meet an individual's health needs, using communication and available resources to promote high-quality, cost-effective outcomes (National Case Management Task Force, 1993).

***Chemical Dependency.** A generic term relating to psychological or physical dependency, or both, on one or more psychoactive substances. No longer in wide use.

Client. The terms "client" and "patient" sometimes are used interchangeably, although staff in medical settings more commonly refer to "patients," while individuals who receive services in nonmedical outpatient settings often are referred to as "clients." (Because addiction is a medical disorder, ASAM prefers the term "patient.")

Clinically Managed Services. Clinically managed services are directed by nonphysician addiction specialists rather than medical personnel. They are appropriate for individuals whose primary problems involve emotional, behavioral, or cognitive concerns; readiness to change, relapse, or recovery environment; and whose problems in Dimension 1 (intoxication/withdrawal) and Dimension 2 (biomedical concerns), if any, are minimal or can be managed through separate arrangements for medical services.

Clinical Necessity. Synonymous with "medical necessity" (see later). Sometimes used to broaden inappropriately narrow definitions of medical necessity.

Coalition for National Clinical Criteria. A multidisciplinary group of individuals involved in alcohol and other drug treatment, research, reimbursement, professional associations, and state and federal government. The Coalition formed in November 1992 to assess support for the adoption of national patient placement criteria and to determine methods of garnering the support of the treatment field for such criteria.

Cognitive-Behavioral Therapy (CBT). CBT is among the most well-studied and empirically supported nonpharmacologic treatments for addiction. Cognitive-behavioral strategies are based on the theory that learning processes play a critical role in the development of maladaptive behavioral patterns. Through CBT, individuals learn to identify and correct problematic behaviors.

Community Reinforcement Approach (CRA). An intensive outpatient therapy, the goal of CRA is to help patients achieve and sustain abstinence long enough to learn new life skills. This approach facilitates patients' engagement in treatment and systematically aids them in gaining substantial periods of abstinence.

Co-Occurring Disorders. Concurrent substance-related and mental or medical disorders. Other terms used to describe co-occurring substance use and mental disorders include dual diagnosis, dual disorders, mentally-ill chemically-addicted (MICA), chemically-addicted mentally-ill (CAMI), mentally-ill substance abusers (MISA), mentally-ill chemically dependent (MICD), co-existing disorders, comorbid disorders, and individuals with co-occurring psychiatric and substance symptomatology (ICOPSS). Use of the term carries no implication as to which disorder is primary and which secondary, which disorder occurred first, or whether one disorder caused the other. (ASAM prefers "co-occurring disorders.")

Continued Service Criteria. In the process of patient assessment, certain problems and priorities are identified as justifying admission to a particular level of care. Continued Service Criteria describe the degree of resolution of those problems and priorities and indicate the intensity of services needed. The level of function and clinical severity of a patient's status in each of the six assessment dimensions is considered in determining the need for continued service.

Continuing Care. The provision of a treatment plan and organizational structure that will ensure that a patient receives whatever kind of care he or she needs at the time. The treatment program thus is flexible and tailored to the shifting needs of the patient and his or her level of readiness to change. (This term is preferred to "aftercare.")

Continuum of Care. An integrated network of treatment services and modalities, designed so that an individual's changing needs will be met as that individual moves through the treatment and recovery process.

***Cross-tolerance.** Tolerance, induced by repeated administration of one psychoactive substance, that is manifested toward another substance to which the individual has not been recently exposed.

***Decriminalization.** Removal of criminal penalties for the possession and use of illicit psychoactive substances.

Dependence. Past editions of the American Psychiatric Association's *Diagnostic and Statistical Manual of Mental Disorders* used the term "addiction." The current edition uses the term "dependence." This has caused confusion among caregivers and policy makers alike. Such confusion loses the important distinction between physical dependence arising from abuse of a drug, and the *physical dependence without addiction* that can and does occur within the context of good medical care (as when a patient prescribed an opioid analgesic for pain becomes physically dependent on the medication). According to the World Health Organization (WHO), "The development of tolerance and physical dependence denote normal physiologic adaptations of the body to the presence of an opioid" (WHO, 1996).

AAPM, APS, and ASAM have agreed on the following definition: "Physical dependence is a state of adaptation that is manifested by a drug class specific withdrawal syndrome that can be produced by abrupt cessation, rapid dose reduction, decreasing blood level of the drug, and/or administration of an antagonist" (AAPM, APS, and ASAM, 2001). ASAM now uses this term only to refer to physical dependence, regardless of the presence or absence of addiction.

This distinction is reflected in the two primary diagnostic classification systems used by health care professionals: the *International Classification of Mental and Behavioural Disorders,*

10th Edition (*ICD-10*; WHO, 1996), and the *Diagnostic and Statistical Manual, Fourth Edition, Text Revision,* of the American Psychiatric Association (*DSM-IV-TR;* APA, 2000). The distinction is observed in this document.

Detoxification. Detoxification (also termed "medically supervised withdrawal") refers to a gradual reduction, or tapering, of the medication dose over time, under the supervision of a physician, to achieve the elimination of tolerance and physical dependence to opioid medications. "Tapering" also is a synonym for these terms. "Detoxification" is a legal and regulatory term that has fallen into disfavor with some in the medical community; indeed, some experts view "detoxification" as a misnomer because many abusable drugs are not toxic when administered in proper doses in a medical environment (Center for Substance Abuse Treatment [CSAT], 2007).

Dimension. A term used in the ASAM *Patient Placement Criteria* to refer to one of six patient problem areas that must be assessed in making a placement decision.

Discharge. The point at which an individual's active involvement with a treatment service is terminated, and he or she no longer is carried on the service's records as a patient.

Dual Diagnosis. Refers to the patient who has signs and symptoms of concurrent substance-related and mental disorders. Other terms used to describe such co-occurring disorders include co-occurring disorders, dual disorders, mentally ill chemically addicted (MICA), chemically addicted mentally ill (CAMI), mentally ill substance abusers (MISA), mentally ill chemically dependent (MICD), coexisting disorders, comorbid disorders, and individuals with co-occurring psychiatric and substance symptomatology (ICOPSS).

Dual Diagnosis Capable (DDC). Describes treatment programs that address co-occurring mental and substance-related disorders in their policies and procedures, assessment, treatment planning, program content, and discharge planning. They have arrangements in place for coordination and collaboration with mental health services. They also can provide psychopharmacologic monitoring and psychological assessment and consultation on site or through coordinated consultation off-site. Staff are capable of addressing the interaction of mental and substance-related disorders and their effect on the patient's readiness to change, relapse, and recovery environment issues. However, the primary focus of a Dual Diagnosis Capable program remains treatment of the patient's substance-related disorder.

Dual Diagnosis Enhanced (DDE). Describes treatment programs that incorporate policies, procedures, assessments, treatment, and discharge planning processes that accommodate patients who have co-occurring mental and substance-related disorders. Mental health symptom management groups are incorporated into addiction treatment. Motivational enhancement therapies specifically designed for those with co-occurring mental and substance-related disorders are more likely to be available (particularly in outpatient settings) and, ideally, there is close collaboration or integration with a mental health program that provides crisis back-up services and access to mental health case management and continuing care. In contrast to Dual Diagnosis Capable services, Dual Diagnosis Enhanced services place their primary focus on the integration of services for mental and substance-related disorders in their staffing, services, and program content.

Early Intervention. Services that explore and address any problems or risk factors that appear to be related to use of alcohol and other drugs and that help the individual to recognize the harmful consequences of inappropriate use. Such individuals may not appear to meet the diagnostic criteria for a substance use disorder, but require early intervention for education and further assessment.

***Enabling.** Any action by another person or an institution that intentionally or unintentionally has the effect of facilitating the continuation of an individual's addictive process.

Facility. The physical structure (building or portions thereof) in which treatment services are delivered.

Failure (as in treatment failure). Lack of progress and/or regression at any given level of care. Such a situation warrants a reassessment of the treatment plan, with modification of the treatment approach. Such situations may require changes in the treatment plan at the same level of care or transfer to a different (more or less intensive) level of care to achieve a better therapeutic response. Sometimes used to describe relapse after a single treatment episode—an inappropriate construct in describing a chronic disease or disorder.

***Familial Alcoholism.** A pattern of alcoholism occurring in more than one generation within a family, due to either genetic or environmental factors, or both.

Family and Couples Therapy. The effects of alcohol dependence are far-reaching and patients' family members and loved ones also are affected by the disorder. By including family members and partners in the treatment process, education about factors that are important to the patient's recovery (such as establishing a substance-free environment) can be conveyed. Family members and partners can provide social support to the patient and can help motivate them to remain in treatment.

***Family Intervention.** A specific form of intervention, involving family members of an alcoholic/addict, designed to benefit the patient as well as the family constellation.

Habilitation. The development, for the first time in an individual's life, of an optimum state of health through medical, psychological, and social interventions (also see Rehabilitation).

Harm Reduction. Policies and programs whose primary goal is to reduce the adverse health, social, legal, and economic consequences of drug use, without necessarily reducing or eliminating such use.

Imminent Danger. Three components constitute imminent danger: (a) a high probability that certain behaviors (such as continued alcohol or drug use or relapse) will occur; (b) the likelihood that such behaviors will present a significant risk of serious adverse consequences to the individual and/or others (as in a consistent pattern of driving while intoxicated); and (c) the likelihood that such adverse events will occur in the very near future.

The concept of imminent danger *does not* encompass all the possible things that may happen, but is restricted to the combination of the three factors listed here. On the other hand, the interpretation of imminent danger should not be restricted to acute suicidality, homicidality, or medical or psychiatric problems that create an immediate, catastrophic risk.

***Impairment.** A dysfunctional state resulting from use of psychoactive substances or mental, emotional, or cognitive problems.

Individualized Treatment. Treatment designed to meet a particular patient's needs, guided by a treatment plan that is directly related to a specific, unique patient assessment.

Intensity of Service. The number, type, and frequency of staff interventions and other services (such as consultation, referral, or support services) provided during treatment at a particular level of care.

Intensive Outpatient Treatment. An organized service delivered by addiction professionals or addiction-credentialed clinicians, which provides a planned regimen of treatment, consisting of regularly scheduled sessions within a structured program, for a minimum of 9 hours of treatment per week for adults and 6 hours of treatment per week for adolescents.

Interdisciplinary Team. A group of clinicians trained in different professions, disciplines, or service areas (such as physicians, counselors, psychologists, social workers, nurses, and certified substance abuse counselors) who function interactively and interdependently in conducting a patient's biopsychosocial assessment, treatment plan, and treatment services.

***Intervention.** A planned interaction with an individual who may be dependent on one or more psychoactive substances, with the aim of making a full assessment, overcoming denial, interrupting drug-taking behavior, or inducing the individual to initiate treatment. The preferred technique is to present facts regarding psychoactive substance use in a caring, believable, and understandable manner.

***Intoxication.** A clinical state marked by dysfunctional changes in physiological functioning, psychological functioning, mood state, cognitive process, or all of these, as a consequence of consumption of a psychoactive substance.

Length of Service. The number of days (for inpatient care) or units/visits (for outpatient care) of service provided to a patient, from admission to discharge, at a particular level of care.

Level of Care. As used in the ASAM *Patient Placement Criteria*, this term refers to a discrete intensity of clinical and environmental support services bundled or linked together and available in a variety of settings.

Level of Function. An individual's relative degree of health and freedom from specific signs and symptoms of a mental or substance-related disorder, which determine whether the individual requires treatment.

Level of Service. As used in the ASAM *Patient Placement Criteria*, this term refers to broad categories of patient placement, which encompass a range of clinical services such as early intervention, detoxification, or opioid maintenance therapy services and levels of care such as intensive outpatient treatment or clinically managed medium intensity residential treatment.

***Loss of Control.** The inability to consistently limit the self-administration of psychoactive substances.

Matching. A process of selecting treatment resources to conform to an individual patient's needs and preferences, based on careful assessment. Matching has been shown to increase treatment retention and thus to improve treatment outcome. It also improves resource allocation by directing patients to the most appropriate level of care and intensity of services.

Medically Managed Treatment. Services that involve daily medical care, where diagnostic and treatment services are directly provided and/or managed by an appropriately trained and licensed physician.

Medically Monitored Treatment. Services that are provided by an interdisciplinary staff of nurses, counselors, social workers, addiction specialists, and other health care professionals and technical personnel, under the direction of a licensed physician. Medical monitoring is provided through an appropriate mix of direct patient contact, review of records, team meetings, 24-hour coverage by a physician, and quality assurance programs.

Medical Necessity. Pertains to essential care for biopsychosocial severity; defined by the extent and severity of problems identified in a multidimensional assessment of the individual.

***Misuse.** Any use of a prescription medication or over-the-counter agent that departs from the prescribed therapeutic regimen or accepted medical practice.

Modality. A specific type of treatment (technique, method, or procedure) that is used to relieve symptoms or induce behavior change. Modalities of addiction treatment include, for example, detoxification or antagonist medication, motivational interviewing, cognitive behavioral therapy, group therapy, social skills training, vocational counseling, and self/mutual help groups.

Motivational Enhancement Therapy (MET). MET is a patient-centered counseling approach designed to help patients resolve their ambivalence about engaging in treatment and stopping substance use. MET employs strategies to evoke rapid and internally motivated change in the patient, rather than guiding the patient stepwise through the recovery process. The techniques used are designed to highlight and help resolve ambivalence about becoming abstinent, and to help move patients along the "stages of change" toward the goal of abstinence.

Outpatient Detoxification. See Ambulatory Detoxification.

Outpatient Service. An organized nonresidential service, delivered in a variety of settings, in which addiction treatment personnel provide professionally directed evaluation and treatment for substance-related disorders.

***Overdose.** The inadvertent or deliberate consumption of a dose much larger than that either habitually used by the individual or typically used in treatment, and likely to result in a serious toxic reaction or death.

Patient. As used in the ASAM *Patient Placement Criteria*, an individual receiving alcohol/other drug treatment. The terms "client" and "patient" sometimes are used interchangeably. (Because addiction is a medical disorder, ASAM prefers the term "patient.")

Partial Hospitalization. A generic term encompassing day, night, evening, and weekend treatment programs that employ an integrated, comprehensive, and complementary schedule of recognized treatments. Commonly referred to as "day treatment," a partial hospitalization program does not need to be attached to a licensed hospital.

Physical Dependence. Physical dependence is a state of adaptation this is manifested by a drug class–specific withdrawal syndrome that can be produced by abrupt cessation or rapid dose reduction of a drug, or by administration of an antagonist.

Placement. Selection of an appropriate level of service, based on assessment of a patient's individual needs and preferences.

***Polydrug Dependence.** Concomitant use of two or more psychoactive substances in quantities and with frequencies that cause the individual significant physiological, psychological, and/or sociological distress or impairment.

Polysubstance Dependence. A *DSM-IV* diagnosis (304.80) reserved for behavior during the same 12-month period in which the individual was repeatedly abusing at least three groups of substances (excluding caffeine and nicotine), but no single substance predominated. Such use met the dependence criteria for substances as a group, but not for any specific substance. (Adapted from the *Diagnostic and Statistical Manual of Mental Disorders, Fourth Edition*, American Psychiatric Association, 1994.)

***Prevention.** Social, economic, legal, medical, and/or psychological measures aimed at minimizing the use of potentially addicting substances, lowering the dependence risk in susceptible individuals, or minimizing other adverse consequences of psychoactive substance use. Primary prevention consists of attempts to reduce the incidence of addictive diseases and related problems in a general population. Secondary prevention aims to achieve early detection, diagnosis, and treatment of affected individuals. Tertiary prevention seeks to diminish the incidence of complications of addictive diseases.

***Problem Drinking.** An informal term describing a pattern of drinking associated with life problems prior to establishing a definitive diagnosis of alcoholism. Also, an umbrella term for any harmful use of alcohol, including alcoholism. ASAM recommends that the term not be used in the latter sense.

Program. An organized system of services designed to address the treatment needs of patients.

Psychotherapy. Individual and/or group psychotherapy can help patients reduce the frequency of alcohol use and the amount of alcohol consumed. *Individual therapy* can be provided in many different types of treatment settings (inpatient, outpatient, or a criminal justice institution); affords privacy (which can help some patients disclose more freely); and allows for more one-on-one time than would be possible in a group setting. *Group therapy* is one of the most common nonpharmacologic interventions used to treat alcohol dependence. Group therapy's primary advantages are that it is economical and allows one health care provider to meet with multiple patients in a given session, it typically costs less than individual therapy, and it has the added bonus of peer support.

Readiness to Change. An individual's emotional and cognitive awareness of the need to change, coupled with a commitment to change. When applied to addiction treatment and particularly assessment Dimension 4, Readiness to Change describes the patient's degree of awareness of the relationship between his or her alcohol or other drug use or mental health problems, and the adverse consequences of such use, as well as the presence of specific readiness to change personal patterns of alcohol and other drug use.

Recognize, Understand, and Apply. The distinction in the criteria is made between an individual's ability to *recognize* an addiction problem, *understand* the implications of alcohol and other drug use on the individual's life, and *apply* coping and other recovery skills in his/her life to limit or prevent further alcohol or other drug use. The distinction is in the difference between an intellectual awareness and more superficial acknowledgment of a problem (recognition) and a more productive awareness of the ramifications of the problem for one's life (understanding), and the ability to achieve behavior change through the integration of coping and other relapse prevention skills (application).

Recovery. A process of overcoming both physical and psychological dependence on a psychoactive substance, with a commitment to sobriety. As used in the ASAM *Patient Placement Criteria*, "recovery" refers to the overall goal of helping a patient to achieve overall health and well-being.

Recovery Environment. As used in Dimension 6 of the ASAM *Patient Placement Criteria*, encompasses the external supports for recovery. The quality and extent of services (such as child care, transportation, crisis and transitional housing, and other "wrap around" services) influence treatment outcome.

*__Rehabilitation.__ The restoration of an optimum state of health by medical, psychological, and social means, including peer group support, for an alcoholic or addict, a family member, or a significant other.

Relapse. Relapse has been variously defined as "a breakdown or setback in a person's attempt to change or modify any target behavior" (Marlatt & Gordon, 1985) and as "an unfolding process in which the resumption of substance abuse is the last event in a long series of maladaptive responses to internal or external stressors or stimuli" (National Institute on Drug Abuse [NIDA], 2005). Relapse rarely is caused by any single factor and often is the result of an interaction of physiologic and environmental factors.

The term *lapse* (sometimes referred to as a *slip*) refers to a brief episode of drug use after a period of abstinence. A lapse usually is unexpected, of short duration, with relatively minor consequences, and marked by the patient's desire to return to abstinence. However, a lapse also can progress to a full-blown relapse, marked by sustained loss of control.

Relapse, Continued Use, or Continued Problem Potential. As used in Dimension 5 of the ASAM *Patient Placement Criteria*, the patient's attitudes, knowledge, and coping skills, as well as the likelihood that the patient will relapse from a previously achieved and maintained abstinence and/or stable and healthy mental health function. If an individual has not yet achieved abstinence and/or stable and healthy mental health function, this dimension assesses the likelihood that the individual will continue to use alcohol or other drugs and/or continue to have mental health problems.

Resident. A patient in one of the clinically managed, residential levels of care.

Setting. A specific place in which treatment is delivered. Settings for alcohol/other drug treatment include hospitals, methadone clinics, community mental health centers, and prisons or jails.

Severity of Illness. Specific signs and symptoms for which a patient requires treatment, including the degree of impairment and the extent of a patient's support networks.

***Sobriety.** A state of complete abstinence from psychoactive substances by an addicted individual, in conjunction with a satisfactory quality of life.

Social Support System. The network of relationships that surround an individual. A health social support system—involving family members, friends, employers, members of mutual support groups, and others—tends to support an individual's recovery efforts and goals. What these individuals have in common is that their relationship with the individual is current and that the individual is comfortable contacting them in times of distress.

Stages of Change. This refers principally to the work of Prochaska and DiClemente, who described how individuals progress and regress through various levels of awareness of a problem, as well as the degree of activity involved in a change in behavior. While their original work studied individuals who changed from smokers to nonsmokers, the concept of stages of change subsequently has been applied to a variety of behaviors.

Substance-Induced Disorders. Includes Substance Intoxication, Substance Withdrawal, and a variety of substance-induced disorders: Delirium, Persisting Dementia, Persisting Amnestic Disorder, Psychotic Disorder, Mood Disorder, Anxiety Disorder, Sexual Dysfunction, and Sleep Disorder. Specific diagnostic criteria are listed in the *Diagnostic and Statistical Manual of Mental Disorders, Fourth Edition* (*DSM-IV*) of the American Psychiatric Association. In the ASAM *PPC-2R*, the term "Substance-Induced Disorder" is used in the diagnostic admission criteria for detoxification services because this diagnostic subgroup is more specific to detoxification than the broader category of Substance-Related Disorders.

Substance-Related Disorders. Includes disorders related to the taking of a drug of abuse (including alcohol), to the side effects of a medication, and to toxin exposure and are divided into two groups: the Substance Use Disorders and the Substance-Induced Disorders, as defined in the *Diagnostic and Statistical Manual of Mental Disorders, Fourth Edition* (*DSM-IV*) of the American Psychiatric Association. In the ASAM *PPC-2R*, the broader diagnostic category of Substance-Related Disorders is used when the criteria involve both diagnostic subgroups. When the criteria relate only to one of the diagnostic subgroups or to a disorder within a subgroup, the specific diagnostic group or disorder is used in the diagnostic admission criteria.

Substance Use Disorders. Includes Substance Dependence and Substance Abuse with specific diagnostic criteria listed in the *Diagnostic and Statistical Manual of Mental Disorders, Fourth Edition* (*DSM-IV*) of the American Psychiatric Association. Substance Use Disorders are one of two subgroups of the broader diagnostic category of Substance-Related Disorders. In the *ASAM PPC-2R*, the specific subgroup or disorder is used in the diagnostic admission criteria, depending on the particular level of care involved. For example, "Substance Dependence" is used for Clinically Managed Medium-Intensity Residential Treatment, Level III.5, because this is not an appropriate level of care for a person who only meets diagnostic criteria for Substance Abuse.

Support Services. Support services are those readily available to the program through affiliation, contract, or because of their availability to the community at large (e.g., 911 emergency response services). They are used to provide services beyond the capacity of the staff of the program and which will not be needed by patients on a routine basis or to augment the services provided by staff.

Tolerance. Tolerance is a state of physical adaptation in which exposure to a drug over time induces changes that result in a diminution of one or more of the drug's effects (AAPM, APS, & ASAM, 2001). For example, tolerance may occur both to an opioid's analgesic effects and to its unwanted side effects, such as respiratory depression, sedation, or nausea. Many characteristics of tolerance remain poorly understood. Most investigators agree that absolute tolerance does not occur.

Transfer. Movement of a patient from one level of service to another, within the continuum of care.

***Treatment.** Application of planned procedures to identify and change patterns of behavior that are maladaptive, destructive, and/or injurious to health; or to restore appropriate levels of physical, psychological, and/or social functioning.

Triage. As used in the ASAM *Patient Placement Criteria,* decision making at the conclusion of an initial assessment process to determine the specific services a patient needs and the level of care at which those services initially should be delivered.

Twenty-Three Hour Observation Bed. Admission for no more than 23 hours for assessment and stabilization to determine the need for inpatient versus outpatient care. Such a "bed" may be located in an inpatient or an outpatient setting (such as a hospital emergency department).

Unbundling. An approach to treatment that seeks to provide the appropriate combination of specific services to match a patient's needs. The goal of unbundling is to provide an array of options for flexible individualized treatment, which can be delivered in a variety of settings. The intensity of clinical services are determined independently of the individual's need for supportive living arrangements and other environmental supports.

***Withdrawal Syndrome.** The onset of a predictable constellation of signs and symptoms following the abrupt discontinuation of, or rapid decrease in, dosage of a psychoactive substance.

REFERENCES

Allen, J. P., & Columbus, M. (1995). *Assessing alcohol problems – A guide for clinicians and researchers.* Bethesda, MD: National Institute on Alcohol Abuse and Alcoholism.

American Academy of Pain Medicine, American Pain Society, & American Society of Addiction Medicine. (2001). *Definitions related to the use of opioids for the treatment of pain: A consensus document from the American Academy of Pain Medicine, the American Pain Society, and the American Society of Addiction Medicine.* Glenview, IL: American Pain Society.

American Psychiatric Association. (1994). *Diagnostic and statistical manual of mental disorders, Fourth Edition (DSM-IV).* Washington, DC: American Psychiatric Press.

American Psychiatric Association. (2001). *Diagnostic and statistical manual of mental disorders, Fourth Edition, Text Revision (DSM-IV-TR).* Washington, DC: American Psychiatric Press.

Betty Ford Institute Consensus Panel. (2007). What is recovery? A working definition from the Betty Ford Institute (special article). *Journal of Substance Abuse Treatment, 33,* 221–228.

Center for Substance Abuse Treatment (CSAT). (2007). *Guidelines for the accreditation of opioid treatment programs, Revised.* Rockville, MD: Substance Abuse and Mental Health Services Administration, July 20.

Marlatt, G., & Gordon, J. R. (1985). *Relapse prevention: Maintenance strategies in the treatment of addictive behaviors.* New York: Guilford Press.

Mee-Lee, D., Shulman, G. D., Fishman, M., et al. (2001). *ASAM patient placement criteria for the treatment of substance related disorders, Second Edition-Revised (ASAM PPC-2R).* Chevy Chase, MD: American Society of Addiction Medicine, Inc.

Morse, R. M., & Flavin, D. K. (1992). The definition of alcoholism. *Journal of the American Medical Association, 268,* 1012–1014.

National Case Management Task Force. (1993). *CCM certification guide, CIRSC/Certified Case Manager.* Rolling Meadows, IL: The Task Force.

National Institute on Alcohol Abuse and Alcoholism. (2007). *Clinician's guide to the treatment of alcohol problems.* Bethesda, MD: National Institutes of Health.

National Institute on Drug Abuse (NIDA). (2005). *Principles of drug addiction treatment: A research-based guide.* NIH Publication # 05-4180. Rockville, MD: NIDA, National Institutes of Health.

Prochaska, J. O., DiClemente, C. C., & Norcross, J. C. (1992). In search of how people change: Applications to addictive behaviors. *American Psychologist, 47,* 1102–1114.

Project MATCH Research Group. (1997). Matching alcoholism treatments to client heterogeneity: Project MATCH posttreatment drinking outcomes. *Journal of Studies on Alcohol, 58,* 7–29.

Rinaldi, R. C., Steindler, E. M., Wilford, B. B., & Goodwin, D. (1988). Clarification and standardization of substance abuse terminology. *Journal of the American Medical Association, 259,* 555–557.

Savage, S. R. (2003). Principles of pain management in the addicted patient. In A. W. Graham, T. K. Schultz, M. F. Mayo-Smith, R. K. Ries, & B. B. Wilford. (Eds.). *Principles of addiction medicine.* (3rd ed.). Chevy Chase, MD: American Society of Addiction Medicine, Inc.

World Health Organization (WHO). (1996). *International classification of mental and behavioral disorders, 10th Edition (ICD-10)* (p. 41). Geneva, Switzerland: WHO.

Zweben, A., Pettinati, H. M., Weiss, R. D., Youngblood, M., Cox, C. E., Mattson, M. E., et al. (2008). Relationship between medication adherence and treatment outcomes: The COMBINE study. *Alcoholism, Clinical and Experimental Research, 32,* 9, 1661–1669.

APPENDIX D

Contributors

EDITOR-IN-CHIEF

Marc J. Fishman, M.D.
Medical Director
Maryland Treatment Centers, and
Assistant Professor
Department of Psychiatry
The Johns Hopkins University School of Medicine
Baltimore, Maryland

EDITORS

George Kolodner, M.D.
Medical Director
Kolmac Clinic
Silver Spring, Maryland
Clinical Professor
Department of Psychiatry
Georgetown University School of Medicine
Washington, District of Columbia

David Mee-Lee, M.D.
Training and Consulting
Davis, California

Gerald R. Shulman, M.A., F.A.C.A.T.A.
Training and Consulting in Behavioral Health
Jacksonville, Florida

Bonnie B. Wilford, M.S.
Executive Director, COPE
Coalition on Physician Education About Substance Use Disorders
Yale University School of Medicine
New Haven, Connecticut

EXPERT ADVISORS

David R. Gastfriend, M.D.
Vice President, Medical Affairs
Alkermes, Inc.
Cambridge, Massachusetts

Henry R. Kranzler, M.D.
Professor of Psychiatry
Department of Psychiatry
University of Connecticut Health Center
Farmington, Connecticut

Edward Nunes, M.D.
Professor of Clinical Psychiatry
New York State Psychiatric Institute
New York, New York

Charles P. O'Brien, M.D., Ph.D.
Kenneth Appel Professor, and
Vice Chair of Psychiatry
University of Pennsylvania
Philadelphia, Pennsylvania

Richard N. Rosenthal, M.D.
Professor of Clinical Psychiatry
Columbia University
College of Physicians & Surgeons, and
Chair, Department of Psychiatry
St. Luke's Roosevelt Hospital Center
New York, New York

Frank J. Vocci, Ph.D.
President, Friend's Research Institute
Baltimore, Maryland

Mark Willenbring, M.D.
Director, Division of Treatment & Recovery Research
National Institute on Alcohol Abuse and Alcoholism
National Institutes of Health
Bethesda, Maryland

Denise E. Greene, M.D.
Medical Director
Kaiser CDRP
Del Rey, California

Mickey Greenfield, J.D., Ph.D., C.A.P.
Executive & Clinical Director
Greenfield Center
Jacksonville, Florida

Raju Hajela, M.D., M.P.H., F.A.S.A.M.
Calgary, Alberta, Canada

Steven S. Kipnis, M.D., F.A.C.P., F.A.S.A.M.
Medical Director
New York State Office of Alcoholism & Substance Abuse Services
Orangeburg, New York

FIELD REVIEWERS

Kay M. Doughty, M.A., C.A.P., C.A.P.P.
Vice President of Family & Community Services
Operation PAR
Pinellas Park, Florida

Kenneth Freedman, M.D., M.B.A., F.A.C.P., F.A.S.A.M.
Chief of Medicine
Lemuel Shattuck Hospital
Boston, Massachusetts

Devang Gandhi, M.D.
Department of Psychiatry
University of Maryland
Baltimore, Maryland

Karen G. Garrett, C.A.P., C.A.P.P., C.M.H.P.
Senior Director
Quality Improvement & Training
River Region Human Services, Inc.
Jacksonville, Florida

Petros Levounis, M.D.
Assistant Professor of Clinical Psychiatry
Columbia University College of Physicians and Surgeons, and
Director, The Addiction Institute of New York
New York, New York

Todd W. Mandell, M.D.
Medical Director
Vermont Office of Drug and Alcohol Programs
Burlington, Vermont

Ken Minkoff, M.D.
Clinical Assistant Professor
Harvard Medical School
Acton, Massachusetts

David Renaud, M.A., L.P.C.
Wyoming Recovery Center
Casper, Wyoming

Melissa Lee Warner, M.D.
Farley Center
Williamsburg, Virginia

Ted Watson
Anderson, South Carolina

Christopher J. Welsh, M.D.
Assistant Professor
Department of Psychiatry
Division of Alcohol & Drug Abuse
University of Maryland School of Medicine
Baltimore, Maryland

Wayne E. Wirta, M.Div.
President and CEO
National Council on Alcoholism and Drug Dependence of New Jersey (NCADD-NJ)
Robbinsville, New Jersey

George E. Woody, M.D.
Director, CRE Team on Addictions/MIRECC
Philadelphia VAMC, and
Treatment Research Institute
University of Pennsylvania
Philadelphia, Pennsylvania

Martha J. Wunsch, M.D.
University of Kentucky
College of Medicine
Lexington, Kentucky

Joan E. Zweben, Ph.D.
Executive Director
East Bay Community Recovery Project
14th Street Clinic
Berkeley, California

COALITION FOR NATIONAL CLINICAL CRITERIA STEERING COMMITTEE

George Kolodner, M.D. (Chair)
Medical Director
Kolmac Clinic
Silver Spring, Maryland
Clinical Professor
Department of Psychiatry
Georgetown University School of Medicine
Washington, District of Columbia

Scott Boyles, L.A.C.
National Association of Alcohol and Drug Abuse Counselors
Helena, Montana

Paul H. Earley, M.D., F.A.S.A.M.
Medical Director
Talbott Recovery Campus

Marc Fishman, M.D.
Medical Director
Maryland Treatment Centers
Assistant Professor
Department of Psychiatry
Johns Hopkins University School of Medicine
Baltimore, Maryland

David R. Gastfriend, M.D.
Vice President
Medical Affairs
Alkermes, Inc.
Cambridge, Massachusetts

John M. Golden, C.D.R., U.S.P.H.S., Ph.D.
Chief of Clinical Practice Consultation
Defense Centers of Excellence for PH & TBI Psychological Health Standards of Care
Department of Defense
Silver Spring, Maryland

Ronald J. Hunsicker, D.Min., F.A.C.A.T.A.
President/CEO
National Association of Addiction Treatment Providers (NAATP)
Lancaster, Pennsylvania

Daniel Kirlahan, Ph.D.
VA Puget Sound Health Case System
Seattle, Washington

Robert Lindsey, M.Ed.
President and CEO
National Council on Alcoholism and Drug Dependence
New York, New York

Eileen McGrath, J.D.
Executive Vice President/CEO
American Society of Addiction Medicine
Chevy Chase, Maryland

David Mee-Lee, M.D. (Past Chair)
Training and consulting
Senior Vice President
The Change Companies
Davis, California

Rob Morrison
Interim Executive Director
National Association of State Alcohol and Drug Abuse Directors
Washington, District of Columbia

Gerald Shulman, M.A., F.A.C.A.T.A.
Training and consulting in behavioral health
8658 Rolling Brook Lane
Jacksonville, Florida

R. James Thatcher, M.D.
Medical Director
Massachusetts Behavioral Health Partnership
Value Options
Boston, Massachusetts

Bonnie B. Wilford, M.S.
Executive Director
Coalition on Physician Education About Substance Use Disorders
Yale University School of Medicine
New Haven, Connecticut

INDEX

Page numbers followed by *f* or *t* indicate material in figures or tables, respectively.

D

E

O

P

R